INTRODUCTION

As a consultant neurosurgeon I have observed that most of the neurosurgical cases have typical presentation and if the resident doctor is well versed with the common symptoms, signs and radiological presentation of the neurosurgical cases, it becomes very easy to diagnose and treat such neurosurgical cases. Although it appears that neurosurgery is a very tough subspecialty of medical sciences, but in fact it is very much predictable and easy to learn. The learning is easy because most of the principles are well understood. As all the functions of the body are anatomically represented in brain and spinal cord so if any part of the brain or spinal cord is affected there will be specific deficit of that part of the body. For example, if there is basal ganglia hematoma on left side of the brain, there will be sudden onset weakness of the right half of body. Similarly, if there is transaction of the spinal cord at the dorsal spine vertebra at D10 level there will be paralysis of both the lower limbs with bladder and bowel involvement. So, diagnosis of the neurosurgical cases can be made with mathematical accuracy, provided a resident doctor is aware about the basics of neurological examination.

So, history taking, general and neurological examination and interpretation of the neuro-radiological examination are the basic knowledge to begin neurosurgery training. So, this book will help you to have bird eye view of practice of neurosurgery. I have deliberately written this guide in brief so that the entire spectrum of neurosurgery can be understood by resident doctors within few hours or days.

Neurosurgery resident doctors face different problems in different clinical settings, OPD, IPD, Operation theatre, Emergency, etc. But understanding of the basic concepts can be applied and time constraints or urgency of approaching neurosurgical cases does not bother a resident doctor. The knowledgeable resident doctors are the backbone of neurosurgical departments as neurosurgery is a very demanding subspeciality of surgery. The senior neurosurgeons and mentors also find difficulty in repeating the instruction in each case. So, this template of neurosurgical guidance will be helpful for all the doctors, whether senior or junior, involved in treating neurosurgical cases.

Practical guide for Resident doctors who treat patients in Neurosurgery Outpatient Department (OPD)

Neurosurgery resident doctors are expected to know the common neurosurgical conditions and their clinical presentations. The common neurosurgical conditions and common neurological symptoms with which majority of patients attend neurosurgery OPD are :

1. Head Injury

2. Brain tumor

3. Hydrocephalus: Post tubercular meningitis (TBM) hydrocephalus, post traumatic, congenital, secondary to intracranial tumor or other space occupying lesions (ICSOL), Benign intracranial cyst

4. Lower Backache, weakness of limbs , numbness in limbs, parasthesia in one or both lower limbs

5. Neck Pain, cervical spondylosis, Craniovertebral junction anomaly, Quadriparesis, weakness in upper limb, weakness of hand grip, atrophy of small muscles of hand, spasticity or stiffness of the body or limbs

6. Seizures, partial seizures, history of loss of consciousness

7. Meningomyelocele, spina bifida

8. Stroke, CVA, TIA, Spontaneous intracerebral hematoma, hypertensive bleed, hemorrhagic stroke

9. Cranial and/or spinal tuberculosis

9. Scalp or skull swelling, Sebaceous cyst, Dermoid, Neurofibroma, Lipoma, osteomyelitis, osteoma

10. Brain or spinal metastasis

The main difference between indoor (in ward, bed side) and outdoor department (OPD) is the paucity of time. So, in OPD it requires ability to obtain brief history and then do clinical examination accordingly. Advise relevant investigations and develop a management plan of the patient including radiological investigations and treatment. The prescription is the evidence of your clinical judgement and approach towards that disease. This OPD card consists of Provisional diagnosis, first investigation, investigation of choice for the particular disease and the appropriate prescription. Patient carries this prescription with him or her which guides the patient, pharmacist, Labortory departments and other doctors and stakeholders. This prescription also guides you, your colleague or consultant when you or someone else sees the patient in follow up OPD. This prescription is carried by the patient and is very frequently shared with many stakeholders.

Although it seems challenging to mention all the details in prescription but with practice it gradually becomes easy. The good part of this process is that it is very often repetitive and you observe a trend and develop your own pattern of seeing patients in OPD.

Learn to take history in brief for OPD and spend few minutes and listen to the complaints of the patient.

Learn neurological examination in the neurosurgery ward and try to emulate that in OPD.

Common investigations which are useful in the management of neurological diseases are:

Hemoglobin, RBC count, PCV(hematocrit), MCHC, PCV, reticulocyte count are useful in the diagnosis of anemia which is a very common cause of headache.

White blood cell count (WBC) for infection

Platelet count for the diagnosis of thrombocytopenia, spontaneous intracranial bleed

Eythrocyte sedimentation rate (ESR) for predicting response to the treatment, or a chronic disease

Bleeding time, clotting time, PT for Pre Anesthetic Check up (PAC) before surgery

Peripheral blood smear for the diagnosis of type of anemia, Malarial parasite

Random blood sugar (RBS), HbAC1 (Diabetes mellitus), kidney function test (KFT), Serum electrolyte, liver function test (LFT), Lipid profile are helpful in diagnosis of patients with stroke and comorbidity.

Thyroid function test: anxiety, depresssion, pituitary adenoma, headache

Urine routine microscopy, urine culture

Serum B12 level, serum vitamin D3 level

CRP, RA factor

Various imaging modalities used for investigating neurological disorders are:

X-Rays (Plain radiography)

Ultrasonography

Carotid doppler

Computerized axial tomography (CAT scan or CT scan) of the brain & Spine, CT scan with contrast, CT Angiography

Magnetic resonance imaging (MRI) Brain and Spine, MR Angiography, MRI with contrast, MR Spectroscopy, MR Tractography, Functional MRI of the brain, MR cisternography

Angiography, Digital substraction angiography (DSA)

Myelography, CT myelogram

PET CT Scan (Positron emission tomography CT scan)

PET MRI

TCD (Transcranial Doppler)

SPECT

Plain Radiography

X-Ray skull is useful for the diagnosis of skull bone osteomyelitis, craniovertebral junction (CV junction) abnormalities. Tumors of the cranial bones like osteomas, osteosarcoma, metastasis to skull may be seen on skull X - ray films. Skull fractures in head injury & Growing skull fractures in children are diagnosed on skull radiography. So, the relevance of skull x-ray is still relevant in some cases, especially in diagnosis of osteomyelitis and growing skull fracture.

CT scan: CT scan is commonly used abbreviation of Computed Axial Tomography (CAT) scanning. This investigation machine was developed in 1970s and it was a most important development in the field of Neuroradiology after the development of X rays (1890s) and angiography (1920s and 1930s). It is a non invasive procedure and uses X-rays for the imaging. It utilizes X-Ray beam which passes through the tissue and produces a picture like x ray but in varying shades of grey. The density of tissue changes the picture. CT scan produces axial or cross sectional (slices) images of the body.
Computer measures the density of the tissue through which x ray beam passes. CT scan machine uses multiple pencil beams of x-ray which rotate in the gantry and pass through the body and on opposite side dosimeter measures the amount of radiation reaching it. Each cubic part of tissue is known as voxel (in new machines about 512 voxels) . Each voxel produces a pixel. Computer measures the attenuation of the beam and assigns a Hounsfield

Unit (HU).

Sir Godfrey Hounsfield from England and Allan McLeod Cormack from USA shared Nobel prize in 1979 for invention of CT scan. All shades of Gray for image May be assigned a number 'HU'. Any HU value below minus 15 will appear pure black on CT film and any HU value above 155 HU will appear pure white. Common HU values are water zero (0) CSF in brain 10 to 16, Air minus 1000, Fat minus 60 to minus 120. Fat containing medullary bone will appear less white as compared to compact cortical bone (HU +1000).

CT scan of the brain is the investigation of choice

For brain trauma patients, because
- it is less time consuming,
- the presence of the metal (bullet in gun shot injury, metal in stab injury) is not a contraindication,
- an trauma patient where the history of pace maker of heart or metallic implant is not known, CT scan is possible,
- detects bony injuries, like a fracture, depressed fracture and hematoma associated with fracture
- better delineation of hematoma.

CT scan brain is also an investigation of choice

For detecting subarachnoid hemorrhage (spontaneous subarachnoid hemorrhage) due to rupture of an intracranial aneurysm

CT angiography (CTA) is an investigation to detect the aneurysm of the brain. It has become an important tool for detecting the site of aneurysm bleed, location, and other characteristics of the aneurysm of the brain. It is more sensitive than MR Angiography and its sensitivity is comparable to the Digital Substarction Angiography.

CT scan of the spine: Although MRI of the spine is undoubtedly the investigation of choice for spine, CT scan of the spine is still an important investigation. CT scan of the spine is required when MRI of the spine is not possible, for example, if a patient is with metal prosthesis (spinal instrumentation with ferromagnetic material like steel), or a metallic bullet is impinged in the spinal cord following a gun shot injury. CT spine also helps in conditions like canal stenosis, bony fractures, ossified posterior longitudinal ligaments, etc.

High resolution CT scan, 3D reconstruction, CT myelogram, Perfusion Coputed Tomography, Intraoperative CT scan are other applications of CT scan.

MRI is the most important development in the field of neuroradiology after the development of X- rays, Angiography, and CT scan.

MRI is a non invasive radiological investigation. It does not expose the patient to the risk of radiation. It uses magnetic field. It provides multiplanar images, i.e, images in sagittal, coronal and axial planes.

Functional MRI is another non invasive investigation which helps in imaging of the eloquent area of the brain.

MR Spectroscopy provides the clue about the nature of the lesion and helps in identifying infective and neoplastic lesions of the brain.

Intraoperative MRI is an advanced technique for intraoperative imaging of the lesions inside the operation theater.

How to interpret MRI brain images?

MRI images are usually black & white. There are T1 weighted, T2 weighted, FLAIR, Diffusion weighted images and if contrast is given then T1 contrast images.

To identify T1 weighted image, see the ventricles. lateral Ventricles are in the center and contain CSF.

On CT usually only Axial images are seen but on MRI Axial, Coronal and sagittal images are seen.

On T1 weighted image, CSF will appear Black (Hypointense).

On T2 weighted image, CSF will appear White (Hyperintense).

On FLAIR (Flow Attenuation Inversion Recovery) the intraventricular CSF will appear Black but brain edema will appear White.

Contrast images are usually T1 contrast Images. So, CSF will appear Black and some lesions like Meningioma will become white (Hyperintense) after contrast enhancement.

PET and SPECT are nuclear neuroimaging and help in physiological assessment. PET (Positron Emission Tomography) is further advanced to utilize CT or MRI imaging techniques and known as PET- CT or PET-MR. PET is used for detecting metastasis and recurrence of the tumor. PET scan commonly utilizes Flurodeoxy glucose (FDG) which is a radioactive tracer.

Digital substraction angiography (DSA) is invasive investigation which involves introducing a catheter and injecting intravenous contrast into the femoral artery. It is the gold standard investigation for defining an intracranial aneurysm, Arteriovenous malformation (AVM) , vasospasm after Subarachnoid hemorrhage (SAH) and other diseases of intracranial vasculature.

TCD (Transcranial Doppler): Non-invasive investigation to detect the vasospasm in a case of SAH.

Although Ultrasound is not a good investigation to detect intracranial pathologies as ultrasound waves do not cross bones, there are certain places where bone is very thin like temporal squama or areas in cranium which have windows like orbit. So, the flow of blood through the intracranial arteries may be detected through these windows. In vasospasm the vessels are narrowed and flow velocity increases. This is the basis of TCD, which is a noninvasive procedure and can be performed on bedside.

Ultrasonography can be used to detect hydrocephalus and meningomyelocele in prenatal period . USG can also detect hydrocephalus in infant as anterior fontanel is not closed.

Intraoperative USG is used for real time imaging , localization, extent of resection of the tumor after craniotomy at the time of neurosurgery.

Neuronavigation is used to localize the lesion, route of the surgery, safer trajectory, etc.

Neurointervention is a very promising development in the field of Neuro-radiology. It is not only useful for the diagnosis but it also offers to treat many ailments of the brain and spine. The most important applications of neurointerventions are: Coiling of the intracranial aneurysms, Preoperative embolization of the vascular tumors like meningioma, Embolization of the intracranial and spinal AVMs, Stenting of the vessel.

HEADACHE

Headache is the commonest symptom and commonest diagnosis among neurological patients.

For Patients coming with complaint of headache which is very common cause of attending neurosurgery OPD, your approach should be very compassionate because patients are most often had already been seen by many doctors.

Pain in head is called headache. Almost everybody experiences headache. One episode of mild headache may be due to exertion, stress or some causes which may not be alarming and you can afford to neglect.

Headache is a very common symptom. Almost everyone experiences headache at some stage of life. Despite of being so common it becomes sometimes it becomes a matter of concern.

So, one should not panic and should analyze the severity of the problem and proceed further for seeking the medical attention & investigations.

Lot of literature is available on the causes of headache but I would like to overly simplify this topic so that one can have an overview.

If headache is associated with exertion at the end of the working day and is over the vertex, frontal or occipital region of the skull and is relieved on taking rest or head massage, one should not worry.

if someone is very stressed and there is obvious stress then there can be **psychogenic headache**. That person should adopt the less stressful lifestyle and practice relaxation exercise , yoga , and very rarely psychotherapy or some medicines may be required.

Maxillary or frontal sinusitis also causes headache.

Redness of eyes, frequent sneezing, cold , allergy may also cause headache. Cluster headache occurs in clusters.

In older persons headache may occur due to hypertension and temporal arteritis.

Refractive errors like myopia and hypermetropia may also cause periorbital pain and headache especially in young children going to school. So vision examination should also be done in patients complaining of headache.

If a child complains of headache it may due to refraction error in vision. Common cause is myopia when someone complains of difficulty in seeing distant things. child may not read the letters written on blackboard in a class and there may be decrease in scholastic performance in school. Another refractive error is hypermetropia which is difficulty in reading the small letters. Although, this is a common problem in people over 40 years of age, it is becoming more common in childrenm because of too much indulgence in mobile games, computer games and less outdoor play activities. So common cause of Persistent headache is refractive error of vision.

Other common cause is sinusitis. Such patients will have frequent history of nasal infections, pain over the bony air sinuses in skull. Maxillary sinusitis, frontal air sinusitis may be diagnosed by tenderness and X-Ray Skull. Sometimes CT scan may be needed. Most of the patients are treated by antibiotics.

Common cause of headache is tension headache. In this type is headache pain is over the vertex, i.e, top of the head. Since the muscles are under continuous tension , such headache will diminish if head massage is given.

Hypertension, anemia may also cause headache.

Migraine is very common and typically paroxysm of throbbing type of headache on irregular intervals, unilateral, associated with vomiting. Migraine is more common in females. There are many variants of migraine.Migraine is the diagnosis of exclusion. Before labelling a ptient with this diagnosis all other causes must be ruled out, like anemia, brain tumor, hemorrhage, infection. CT scan or MRI of the brain rules out any intracranial mass occupying lesion. It is normally hemicranial,i.e., involes one half of the head. It is usually throbbing headache and associated with nauses and vomiting. Migraine is recurrent and gradually the duration between episodes become less.

What should not be missed?

Any physician or person should not ignore headache due to brain tumor and subarachnoid hemorrhage due intracranial aneurysm rupture.

How to recognize headache due to brain tumor? Usually progressive, associated with vomiting, temporarily relieved after vomiting, may be associated with blurring of vision (due to papilloedema), or other neurological deficit.

How to recognize headache due to subarachnoid hemorrhage caused by rupture of intracranial aneurysm? It is sudden onset severe headache (bolt from blue, thunderclap headache which a patient in the age group of 4th - 5th decade, says that he or she had never experienced such type of headache in life time. Sometimes headache may not be so severe and it is called warning leak. There may be associated neck rigidity.

What is the most valuable investigation in the management of headache??

If Visual examination of the patient is performed and Non contrast CT scan of the head is advised one will never be guilty of missing a life threatening brain condition like SAH (subarachnoid hemorrhage and brain tumor) and it will guide the further course of treatment.

Sudden onset severe headache in a person of about 40 to 50 years of age which is so intense as patient describes that he or she had never experienced such headache in his or her life time,"*Bolt from Blue*," is typical of spontaneous subarachnoid hemorrhage (SAH) due to rupture of intracranial aneurysm.

Head trauma, cervical spondylosis may also cause headache.

Headache associated with seizures is alarming. CT scan or MRI of the brain must be done.

HEAD INJURY

If a patient of head injury comes to OPD, you should ask for the mode, manner, time of injury, initial prersentation, initial condition, initial treatment, concussion, post traumatic amensia, seizures, Ear Nose or Throat (ENT) bleed, vomiting, any extracranial injury. You advise NCCT head which is the investigation of choice for diagnosis of head injury.

Concussion means transient loss of consciousness due to head injury.
Concussion is also known as Mild Traumatic Brain Injury (MTBI).
It may be described as alteration of consciousness without structural damage as a result of head trauma.

It is transient loss of consciousness or alteration in mental status like alteration in conscious level, disturbance of vision or balance due to head injury.

Trauma to the head may cause sudden linear or rotational movement of the brain. This sudden acceleration and deacceleration movements of the brain and brain stem disrupts the normal cellular activities in the brain (including fornix, corpus callosum, temporal lobe, frontal lobe) and in the the reticular activating system of the midbrain.

Most of the non medical people use word coma to describe a patient who is unconscious. But for a medical professional word "coma" is very specific because the impairment of arousal can vary from drowsiness (sleepiness) to non-responding to any stimulus like sound or pain. Coma is the severest impairment of arousal, and is defined as the inability to obey commands, speak, or open the eyes to pain.

One should learn the GCS scale to better understand the different levels of impairment of conscious level and to avoid descrepencies in describing the daily condition of the patient by different medical professionals and nurses.
Teasdale and Jennet, in year 1875, proposed a scale known as GCS (Glasgow Coma Scale). Three types of stimulus and response to the patient to these three stimuli is described.

First is EYE OPENING

If patient opens his eyes spontaneously, i.e., like a normal person without any problem, then 4 point is mentioned.

Next situation is that patient is drowsy or feeling sleepy and is having closed eyes. The sleepy patient if opens eyes on sound then 3 point is given.

If patient eyes are closed and he opens eyes only when painful stimulus is given the, only 2 points is given.

And patient does not open eyes even on a painful stimulus then only 1 point is given so the lowest score of eye opening is 1.

E 4 spontaneous eye opening
E 3 opening eyes to speech
E 2 opening eyes to pain
E 1 None

Then patient's verbal response is examined (V stands for verbal response)

V 5   Person is oriented
(aware about what is happening around, Person is oriented to place, person and time)

V 4   Confused or disoriented

V 3   speaking inappropriate words
(Not producing sentences)

V 2   producing incomprehensible words
(Not producing word i.e. only some sound is produced by the patient)

V 1   None (No verbal output means patient is not speaking and even not producing any sound)

Patient's Motor response is assessed

M 6 Obeys
(Best motor resonpse is M6 when patients moves limbs themselves and obey the command to move hand and feet whenever asked to do so)

M 5 patient localizes pain
(when patient is pinched he tries to remove your fingers)

M 4 Withdraws to pain
(here when patient is pinched feels pain and tries to withdraw from the pain)

M 3 Flexion to pain (decorticate)
(in medical terminology it is known as decorticate posture , i.e., posture seen in an animal when the central nervous system is cut just below the level of cerebral cortex. Like in an experient by Sherrington, father of modern neurophysiology, when the brain of a cat was cut just above the midbrain or brain stem, animal,s upper limbs were flexed and lower limbs were extended. This abnormal posture is known as DECORTICATE POSTURE)

M 2 Extensor (decerebrate)
(extensor response to a painful stimulus is a very bad neurological sign. When a patient is pinched his both upper and lower limbs are extended)

M 1 No response to the painful stimulus

The best responses of the patient are added . So, the maximum GCS score is 15 and minimum is 3.

Glasgow coma scale score of equal or less than 8 is a generally accepted operational definition of coma.

It can result from dysfunction of brain stem, diencephalon or lesions of both cerebral hemispheres. This may be due to neoplastic lesions, electrolyte imbalance, metabolic or endocrine problems, vascular lesions, infections, trauma or nutritional reasons.

GCS is an important method of describing patient's neurological condition but blood pressure, pulse rate, respiratory rate, response of the pupils of eye to light, paralysis of the limbs are other important parts of the complete neurological assessment.

Although, concussion is considered as mild head injury but sometimes it has sequelae. Headache, confusion, amnesia, blurring of vision, dizziness, fatigue may persist for some time. More alarming long term sequelae are the cognitive impairment, sleeplessness, difficulty in concentration, irritability, anger, behavioral abnormalities, or maladjustment in the work or studies.

Plain CT scan of brain is the investigation of choice. It is normal in cases of concussion because it is a physiological impairment and so, no anatomical abnormality is seen on non-contrast CT scan of the brain. MRI of the brain is not required and is unnecessary. MRI will demonstrate abnormalities in up to 25% of cases where CT is normal. But, I do not suggest MRI in cases of concussion because CT actually guides the treatment. So, if CT is normal there is nothing serious and no active neurosurgical treatment is required. MRI just adds to the apprehension of the patients and their relatives and it does not provide any additional information of any use to the neurosurgeon.

Symptoms usually resolve in approximately two weeks. But, symptoms may persist for longer period.

Every person with post traumatic concussion requires emotional support. Patient's caregivers, family members, teachers and co-workers and colleagues must understand that some symptoms like irritability, headache, dizziness may be sequelae of concussion. So, a sympathetic and considerate attitude should be adopted towards the person who had suffered mild head injury with concussion and is experiencing long term sequelae of mild head injury.

Symptomatic treatment of like dizziness may be trated with Betahistine or Cinnarazine. Headache is a common complaint and requires both medical and psychological support.

Neurotrophic vitamins like vitamin B complex, Methylcobalamin, vitamin E are useful. Anxiety, sleeplessness are very well managed with tablet Clonazepam 0.25 mg at night and Psychological support.

ABNORMALITIES OF THE CRANIO-VERTEBRAL JUNCTION

Cranio-Vertebral Junction (CV Junction) is the bony junction of the skull and vertebral column. It is formed by Clivus, Occipital bone and C1 and C2 vertebra.

This area is important as any abnormality in this area may lead to compression over the cervico- medullary junction, which is the junction of the cervical region of the spinal cord qnd medulla oblongata.

The abnormality at this region could be congenital anomaly or acquired.

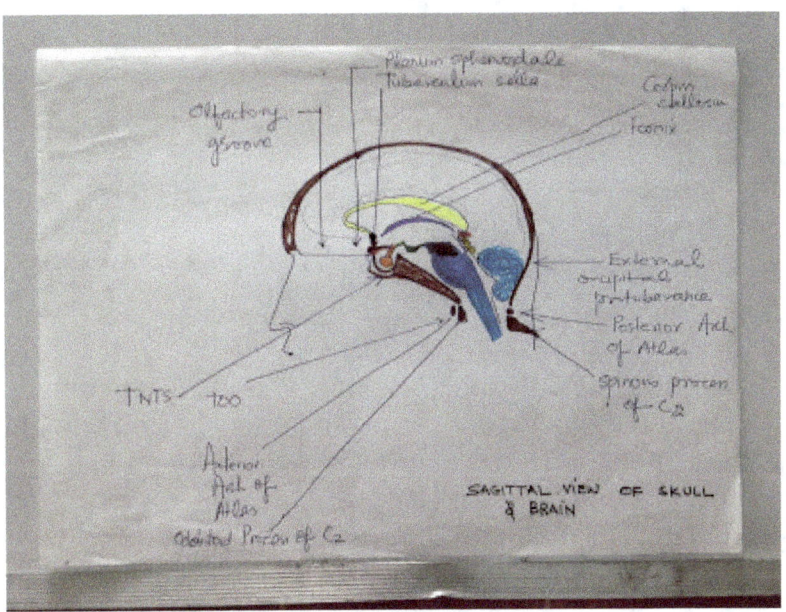

This is simple diagram of the sagittal view shows location of CV Junction. TOO is abbreviation for transoral odontoidectomy . This surgery is done through oral cavity . Anterior arch of Atlas vertebra (first cervical vertebra) lies just anterior to the odontoid process of Axis vertebra (2nd cervical vertebra). Any dislocation of Atlanto-Axial Joint (Atlanto axial dislocation -AAD) may compress over the medulla Oblongata, which lies just posterior to the Dens of the C2 vertebra.

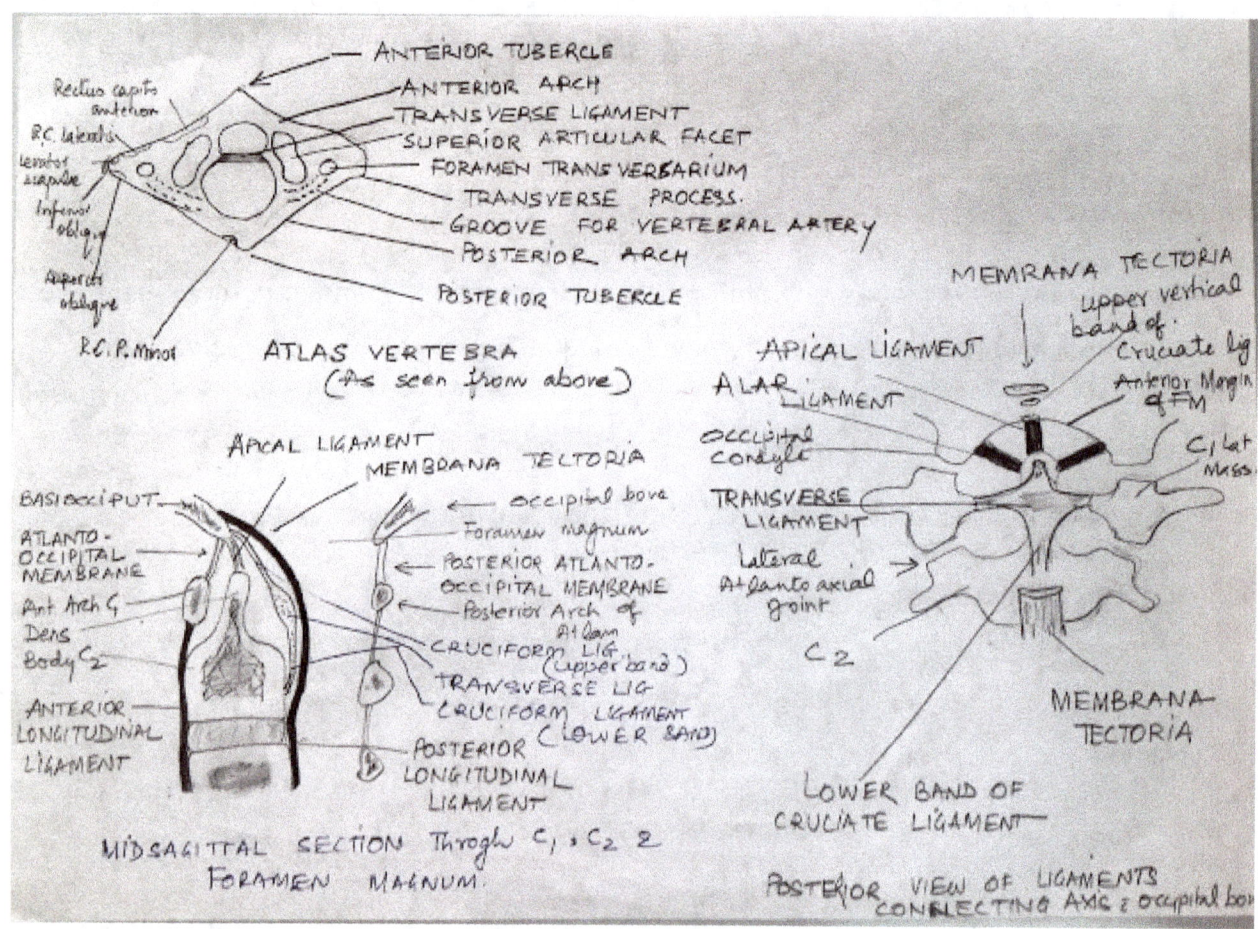

Stability of the CV junction is mainly due to ligaments.

The anterior atlanto-occipital membrane is the cranial extension of the anterior longitudinal ligament. It extends from anterior margin of foramen magnum to anterior arch of C1.

Posterior Atlanto-occipital membrane connects posterior margin of the foramen magnum to the posterior arch of Atlas.

Tectorial Membrane is the upward continuation of posterior longitudinal ligament. It connects the dorsal surface of the Dens of the Odontoid process of C2 vertebra anterior lip of the Foramen magnum.

Apical odontoid Ligament connects the tip of Dens to the anterior lip of Foramen Magnum.

Alar Ligament connects side of the Dens to occipital condyles.

Transverse Ligament is the horizontal component of the Cruciate ligament which traps or straps or binds the Dens anteriorly against the C1. It is the strongest ligament.

INTRACRANIAL BENIGN DEVELOPMENTAL CYSTS

Arahnoid cysts and Ependymal cysts

It is very common observation in brain imaging to find small cysts inside the brain. These cystic areas resemble and look like areas of the brain with normal cerebrospinal fluid. Such incidental finding increase anxiety in the person in whom brain imaging was usually done for some other purpose. Such cysts are usually arachnoid cysts or ependymal cysts.

Arachnoid Cysts

Arachnoid cyst is a benign intracranial developmental cyst which is between two split layers of arachnoid and it usually contains clear colurless CSF.

So, arachnoid cyst is a cyst containing CSF and it forms due to splitting of the archnoid membrane. These are benign congenital malformation.

It is usually an incidental finding.

They are commonly seen in Sylvian fissure, cerebellopontine angle, supracollicular area, vermian area, sellar and suprasellar area, etc. This may appear at any age from infancy and adolescence to adults.

Arachnoid cyst may remain asymptomatic throughout life, only to be diagnosed incidentally by a neuroimaging study. Imaging often shows remodelling of bone, and imaging characteristics exactly mimic CSF on CT and MRI in most cases.

Symptoms and signs of arachnoid cyst depend on its size and location inside the brain and spinal cord.

Recommendation for incidentally discovered arachnoid cyst in adults: a single follow up imaging study in 6-8 months is usually adequate to rule-out any increase in size. Subsequent studies only if concerning symptoms develop.

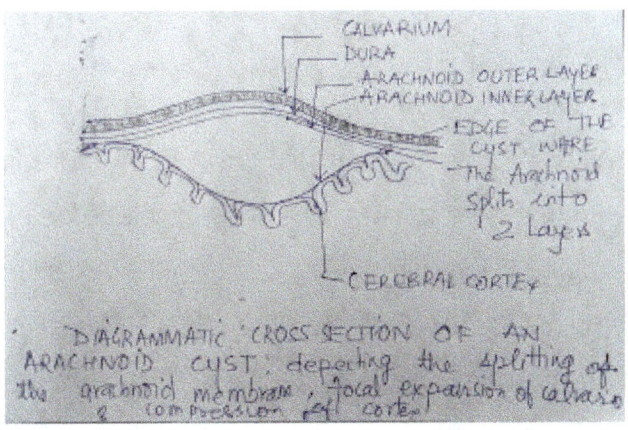

Diagrammatic cross section of an arachnoid cyst depicting the splitting of the arachnoid membrane, focal expansion of calvaria & compression of cortex.

Sylvian fissure archnoid cyst may present with headache, seizures, dysarthria (speech problem), focal bulge in temporal region, exophthalmos, papilloedema, and hemiparesis. X-ray skull or CT scan may show evidence of expansion of the middle cranial fossa, elevation of the lesser wing of the sphenoid, forward protrusion of the greater wing the sphenoid bone and outward expansion and thinning of the temporal bone. But expansion of skull in relation to arachnoid cyst is not an indication for surgery, but mass effect, displacement of midline structures and presence of obsructive hydrocephalus are indications for surgical intervention for middle fossa arachnoid cysts.

On CT, arachnoid cyst appear as low density, smooth bordered lesions having attenuation values similar to that of CSF. The cyst wall has well-defined margins and does not enhance after intravenous injection of contrast agent.

MRI is better at demonstrating multiplanar relationship and characteristics of the lesion on T1, T2, FLAIR, Diffusion weighted images and contrast, MTR (Magnetization transfer ratio), MRS (MR spectroscopy), MRA (MR angiography)study. It helps in differentiating arachnoid cyst from epidermoid, dermoid, lipoma, ependymal cysts, tumors like low grade glioma & metastasis, old hemorrhage, cavernoma, hydatid cyst, hemangioma, and infective granulomas.

On T1 weighted image arachnoid cyst appears hypointense and on T2 weighted image it appears hyperintense like CSF. On T1 weighted MRI, lipomas will appear hyperintense as fat appears hyperintense on both T1 and T2 weighted images.

The high protein content of a nonhemorrhagic tumour cyst will cause the cyst to appearslightly hyperintense to CSF on proton density images. The associated peritumoural oedema of cystic astrocytoma will look hyperintense on FLAIR image of MRI.

Ependymal cysts and epidermoid tumors appear isointense or slightly hyperintense to CSF on proton-density images. Epidermoid tumors are more likely to be lobulated, have less distinct margins, and encase rather than displace neighbouring structures. Diffusion-weighted imaging reflects the amount of Brownian motion of proteins which is greater in cystic than in solid lesions.

Sylvian fissure is the most common site for intracranial arachnoid cysts. Sylvian fissure arachnoid cyst may be of three types. It may be a small lenticular lesion at the anterior pole of the middle cranial fossa without any mass effect (Type 1) or quadrangular in shape reflecting a completely open insula (Type II). Type III sylvian fissure arachnoid cyst presents as large rounded area with significant compression of the brain. Displacement of the midline structures in type III cysts is an indication for surgical decompression.

Treatment of archnoid cyst

Adults with asymptomatic arachnoid cyst should be treated conservatively, even for large cysts without symptoms and signs or with only a complaint of headache. Only arachchnoid cysts which cause a mass effect or neurological deficit should be treated surgically.

In children, decompression of sylvian fissure archnoid cyst is more likely to lead to decreased parenchymal compression, cyst collapse, and subsequent resolution if intracranial hypertension and neurological deficits.

Ventriculoperitoneal shunting

Cystoperitoneal shunting

Cyst fenestration

Cyst excision

Skull may be very thin and may be even eggshell-like, so care must be taken in placing burrhole during surgery. The dura is bluish because of presence a large pool of fluid underneath. The exposed cyst wall may be clear and transparent; in some areas a web of milky thickening may be noted as a result of collagen reinforcement. The forntal lobe appears widely separated from the temporal lobe because of the failure of opercula to develop. So, the insula and branches of middle cerebral artery may be completely exposed after excision of the sylvian fissure arachnoid cyst. When the outer wall of the cyst is excised, clear CSF escapes. Long bridging veins may be observed either on the surface of the cyst or within the cyst. Bridging veins that traverse the cavity of the cyst do not have much support. Rupture of such unsupported veins account for high incidence of subdural hematoma associated with these cysts.

Fenestration of deep wall of cyst creates a communication between the sylvian fissure cyst and the chiasmatic cistern.

A significant number of middle cranial fossa arachnoid cysts are associated with bleeding hematomas which are usually venous in nature and result from tearing of bridging veins within or external to the cyst. It may precipitate symptoms in a previously asymptomatic patient.

Arachnoid cyst in sella turcica

Sella turcica arachnoid cyst may be intrasellar or suprasellar. Suprasellar cysts are by far the more common. It may present with hydrocephalus, visual impairment, endocrine dysfunction (hypopituitarism, stunted growth, etc), gait disturbance. A curious head nodding motion described as the " bobble-head doll syndrome" has been described in suprasellar arachnoid cyst. The nodding or bobbing consists of irregular involuntary head motions in the anteroposterior direction occurring two to three times per second. The motion is reminiscent of that seen in dolls with a weighted head resting on a coiled spring; hence the name of this syndrome. Some degree of mental retardation is associated with this syndrome.

Treatment of suprasellar sella turcica arachnoid cysts are ;endoscopic ventriculostomy with concomitant fenestration of lamina terminalis, subfrontal cyst excision with communication to the basal cisterns, and transcallosal or transventricular cyst excision with concomitant cystoperitoneal shunting.

Treatment of intrasellar sella turcica arachnoid cysts is trans-sphenoidal approach with packing of sella with fat or fascia or muscle tissue.

Arachnoid cysts in Interhemispheric Fissure

Two types of arachnoid cysts occur near the midline in the supratentorial space.

1. Interhemisheric cysts with associated partial or complete corpus callosal agenesis. It straddles the falx and extends equally on either side, compressing the medial surface of both hemispheres. A coronal MRI shows a " bat-wing" appearance of the lateral horns and dorsal displacement of the third ventricle.

2. Parasagittal cysts are usually not associated with agenesis of the corpus callosum. The cyst is strictly unilateral and is sharply limited by falx in the midline, thus it tends to be wedge shaped. There is a marked bulging of the frontal and parietal bones in the parasagittal area. The superior sagittal sinus and falx cerebri are considerably off the midline.

Cerebral convexity arachnoid cyst

In infants, it may present with progressive asymmetrical enlargement of head. MRI findings may mimic subdural hygroma, but without an enhancing membrane
In adults, the lesion may present with seizures, headache , papilloedemaand progressive contralateral hemiparesis. Skull films may show erosion of the inner table of the skull. CT scan shows biconvex or semicircular area of lucency over the

convexity without an enhancing membrane. Surgical therapy consists of excision of the outer membrane of the cyst.

Quadrigeminal cistern arachnoid cysts

These cysts behave like pineal masses and present with hydrocephalus and Parinaud's syndrome. Therapy consists of excision of the cyst wallthrough an occipital transtenorial approach, with or without insertion of cystoperitoneal shunt.

Cerebellopontne angle arachnoid cysts

Clinical presentation of arachnoid cyst in CP angle may mimic that of an acoustic neuroma.

Posterior fossa arachnoid cysts

Posterior fossa arachnoid cysts may present in the midline near the fourth ventricle or the cistrna magna, or paramedian area opposite the cerebellar hemisphere. X-ray skull may show a focal expansion of the occipital bone. Diffrential diagnosis of midline posterior fossa arachnoid cyst include mega cistern magna, Dandy-Walker malformation, epidermoid cyst, cystic glioma and hemangioblastoma.

Clival region arachnoid cysts

The clival region is uncommon site for intracranial arachnoid cyst. Although termed clival , the cyst may extend into the interpeduncular cistern or the cerebellopontine angle. The cyst displaces the midbrain and pons dorsally along with basilar artery.The cranial nerves are stretched , elongated , and draped around the cyst. Other rare locations of arachnoid cysts are intraventricular, diploic space, etc.

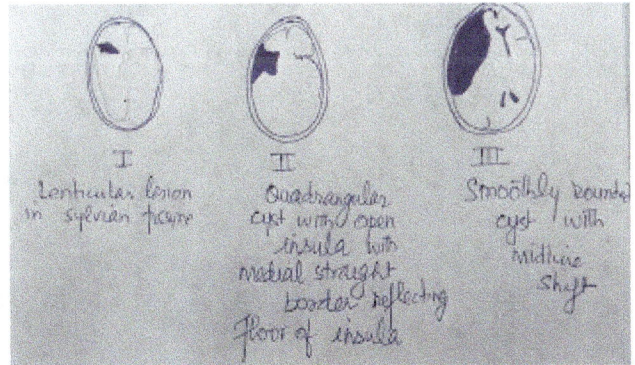

Diagrammatic representation of 3 types of Sylvian fissure arachnoid cyts

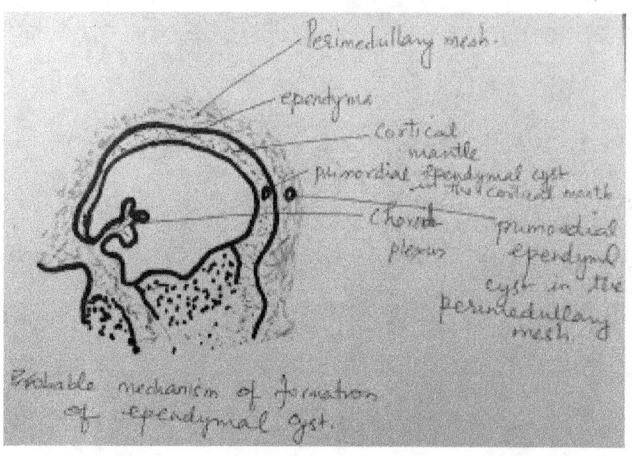

Diagrammatic representation of probable mechanism of formation of ependymal cyst

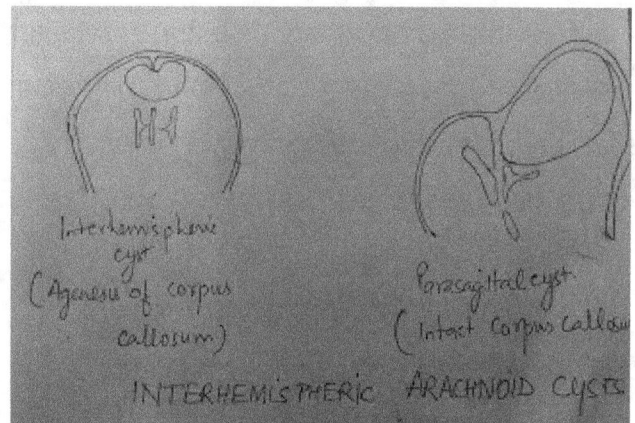

Two types of interhemisheric arachnoid cysts

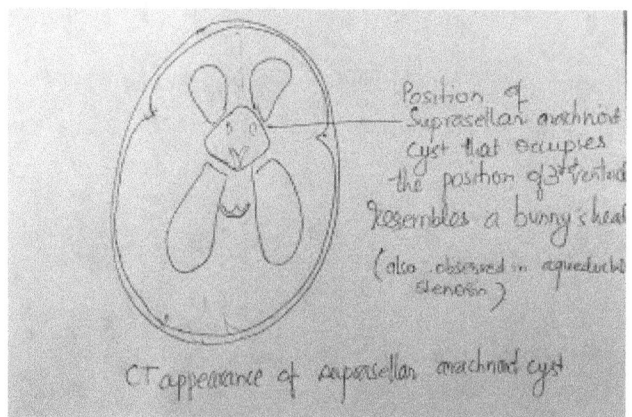

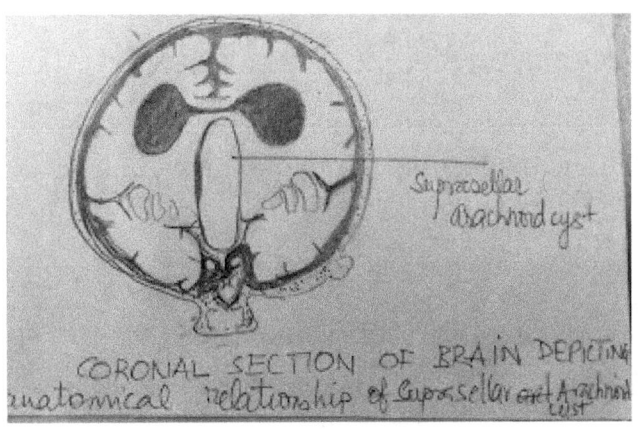

CORONAL SECTION OF BRAIN DEPICTING anatomical relationship of Suprasellar arachnoid cyst

Ependymal cysts

Ependymal cysts may mimic arachnoid cyst clinically and on imaging studies. They occur much less frequently than arachnoid cysts. They occur in central white matter of the frontal and temoporopatrietal lobes, causing progressive neurological deficits, seizures and features of raised intracranial pressure. The protein content of the cyst fluid is generally greater than that of the CSF; on MRI the cyst will typically appear isointense or slightly hyperintense to CSF on proton density images. The wall is lined by columnar or cuboidal cells with or without cilia. Blepharoplasts may or may not be identifiable , These cysts never communicate with the ventricular system. They are believed to arise by the sequestration of a small segment of the primitive ependymal lining into either the cortical mantle or the perimedullary mesh . treatment consists of drainage of the cyst and excision of its wall.

Sources

Neurosurgery, second edition, volume III Editors: Robert H.Wilkins and Setti S.Rengachary, McGraw –Hill, Chapter 374; Intracranial arachnoid and ependymal cysts by Setti S. Rengachary and Jerome D.Kennedy, pages 3709-3728

Wikipedia

Handbook of neurosurgery , Mark S Greenberg, 7th edition, Thieme

SPINA BIFIDA (SPINAL DYSRAPHISM)

Spinal dysraphism means a spectrum of congenital anomalies of the spine and spinal cord.

Spina bifida is a common form of spinal dysraphism. The term spina bifida includes a wide variety of anomalies.

Congenital defect in the spine leads to spina bifida. This can be of two types: spina bifida occulta and spina bifida aperta.

In spina bifida aperta; visible lesion, like a swelling over the midline of the back may be noticed at the time of birth of a child. Such spinal dysraphism is known as Spinal Bifida Aperta.

But, a child may be having some abnormality of the spine or spinal cord but without any externally visible lesion and overlying skin is intact, then it is known as spina bifida occulta. This defect of the vertebrae of the spine of a child may not be visible at the time of birth and there may be no visible exposure of meninges or neural tissue. And, there may be congenital defect only in the lamina of the vertebrae of the spine without any involvement of underlying spinal cord. This is known as spine bifida occulta.

But, in spina bifida aperta there is a visible or open defect in the spine. There may be congenital defect in vertebral arches with cystic distension of meninges which is filled with CSF and is known as Meningocele. If, in this congenital defect of the vertebral arches there is a cystic dilatation of meninges and cerebrospinal fluid along with neural tissue or spinal cord (Myelon) , then it is known as Myelomeningocele. If Myelomengocele contains fat tissue, then it is known as Lipomyelomengocele.

Myelomeningocele is one of the congenital open neural tube defect present at the birth on the back of the newborn.

It is a common type of congenital defect of the spine and its incidence is about 1 in 1,000 live births. Better nutrition and folic acid supplementatiion during the antenatal care of the mother decrease its occurrence.

Ultrasound study during the early antenatal care detects any occurrence of myelomeningocele in a fetus during pregnancy.

A newborn child should be assessed for any sensory or motor deficit due to meningocele or myelomeningocele. There may be associated congenital lesions, like cardiac lesions. Myelomeningocele may be associated with congenital hydrocephalus. So, MRI of the spinal cord and brain is investigation for choice for assessing a case of meningocele. MRI may show whether a swelling on the back of a child is only flled with CSF or does it contain any neural tissue. It detects any intraspinal extension, associated intraspinal dermoid, lipoma, dermal sinus, spina bifida, spinal dysrahism like duplication of the cord, any bony spur between the duplicated cord, Chiari malfomation, syrinx, hydrocephalus, thickened filum terminale, etc. So, MRI helps in diagnosis, surgical planning and predicting prognostic outcome.

COLLOID CYST

Colloid cysts are slow growing benign intraventricular tumor of anterior third ventricle. These constitute less than 1% of all intracranial tumors. It constitutes 14% of intraventricular tumors. It is commonest third ventricular tumor.

It is presumed that it originates from roof of third ventricle from rudimentary paraphysis (evagination in roof of 3rd ventricle during development). It comprises of fibrous epithelial lined cyst filled with either mucoid or gelatinous or dense hyloid substance.

It is commonly seen in between age groups 20 and 40 years. Colloid cyst is usually located in the anterior third ventricle, at the level of foramen of Monro. It may block the cerebrospinal fluid (CSF) flow causing symmetrical dilatation of both lateral ventricles and obstructive hydrocephalus. It may present insidiously or suddenly. Headache is a common presentation. Intermittent and postural nature of attacks are other common type of presentation. Drop attack due to sudden weakness of lower limbs with headache is also commonly seen in patients with colloid cyst.

Other common symptoms of colloid cyst are diplopia, gait disturbance, vomiting, disturbed mentation, blurred vision, incontinence, and vertigo or dizziness. Occurrence of intermittent symptoms is chracteristic of colloid cyst.

CT scan or MRI with contrast is able to detect a rounded lesion in the anterior third ventricle. Most clinicall significant cysts are more than 1.5 centimeter is size. It may show minimal enhancement or no enhancement on CT or MRI. So, the enlargement of both lateral ventricles and sparing of third and fourt ventricle along with a small globular intraventricular lesion at the level of Foramen of Monor should establish the diagnosis of colloid cyst.

Image 1: CT scan of the brain showing axial view of brain with a hyperdense lesion in the anterior third ventricle with enlargemtnt of both lateral ventricles.

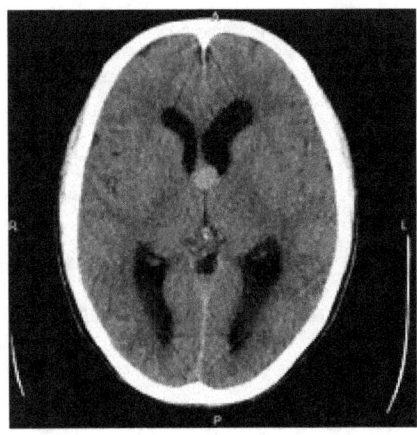

Neurosurgery is the definitive treatment. Lumbar Puncture (LP) is contraindiacated due to risk of herniation. It should be treated surgically as there is risk of acute hydrocephalus and sudden neurological deterioration. Open transcranial surgery or endoscopic neurosurgery are the treatment options. Transcranial surgery may be transcallosal or transcortical. Endoscopic neurosurgical excisison is the mainstay of treatment.

Trancortical approach involves reaching the third ventricle through right sided middle frontal gyrus. It is feasible when ventricles are enlarged.

Transcallosal approach involves approach to the 3rd ventricle either via the foramen of Monro or by interfornicial approach. This approach can be used even if ventricles are not enlarged. There is risk of venous infarction or fornicial injury in this approach.Injury to the fornix is associated with memory deficits or behaviour abnormalities.

Reference

1. Handbook of Neurosurgery by Mark S Greenberg 7th Deition, Thieme publication
2. https://en.wikipedia.org/wiki/Colloid_cyst
3. *radiopaedia.org*

BRAIN METASTASIS

About twenty five years back, as a medical student, I used to feel pity about anybody who was diagnosed with brain tumour, as I thought that all brain tumour patents had dismal prognosis. But, now as a neurosurgeon in year 2018, I understand and know that some brain tumours have favourable surgical outcome and carry good prognosis. Any, very often surgery for the brain tumour is very rewarding for the doctor as well as for the patients and their family members. Like, a patient with large frontal convexity meningioma can be operated safely and whole tumour can be excised without any need for chemotherapy or radiotherapy. So, the patient as well as the neurosurgeon are happy with the favourable outcome. This happiness is sustained even several years after the surgery as there may be no chance of recurrence due to complete excision.

So, as a medical student with initial posting in clinical departments I was like a lay person, observing the plight of patients and their relatives, I was pessimistic about this disease. However, about 13 years ago during my neurosurgical training, I had experienced similar feelings for patients with brain metastasis. I thought that if cancer has spread to the brain of the patient, there would be very bad prognosis. Initially as a trained neurosurgeon I fad operated few patients with that notion, but his presumption was misfounded. Because, there were good prognosis in few patients of brain metastasis.

So, one reason for writing this article is to share my optimism and enthusiasm of managing patients with brain metastasis.

Another reason for writing this topic is to bring to the notice of readers about all available resources for the appropriate and tailor made approach to treat effectively any patient diagnosed with brain metastasis. Because, many medical professionals may not be aware about the favourable outcome in some patients with metastases to the brain.

Last reason is very simple. Most common brain tumour, definitely requires maximum attention. Such lesions with worst prognosis is a challenge and demands amalgamation of all available therapeutic modalities for providing best possible benefits to the patient.

The development of new diagnostic tools and therapeutic interventions in last two decades must be channelized and focussed on managing such cases, so the prognosis of brain metastasis becomes very good. This can be achieved now. If not now, atleast in next few years. This article is an attempt to achieve good neurosurgical outcome of patients with brain metastasis.

Brain metastasis is the commonest brain tumour in adults as almost all cancers metastasize to the brain. A lot to be explored to understand about the disease process, early detection and effective treatment of this disease. With use of even the best available technologies, many patients die of this illness without diagnosis. In many patients brain metastasis is detected at the time of autopsy.

Although, many institutions are equipped with advanced machines and have good infrastructure for managing primary systemic cancers, but very few are having facility to treat cases with brain metastases. It may in part, due to preconception among physicians about the presumption that any patient harbouring multiple metastases has dismal chances of survival. So, to change the conception a paradigm shift is required. This manuscript may be a precursor for much mor clinical works in this field and will guide clinicians for managing a patient with brain metastasis.

Many advances have occurred in past few decades leading to better understanding of this disease. But, there is need to converge the outcome of different basic research , translational research, diagnostic studies and clinical studies of different specialities for the concerted effort to treat brain metastasis. Approach of all stakeholders who are involved in basic, paraclinical and clinical study and management should not be egocentric , but patient centric. These patients require multidisciplinary care . Multidiscilinary approach will definitely advance our understanding about biologyof brain metastasis, different therapeutic options , application of newer diagnostic tools and tailor made approach for managing each and every patient with brain metastasis. Contributions of basic science researcher and people involved in palliative care are equally important.

Brain metastasis is a major cause of morbidity and mortality in patients with systemic malignancies. Newer imaging and treatment modalities have improved clinical outcome in last few decades.

In last 50 years, there has been nearly a five-fold increase in the overall prevalence of brain metastases; the ratio between metastatic to primary brain tumor is now almost 50:50 . The incidence of metastases is rising due to early detection by advanced neuroimaging modalities and effective treatment regimens of systemic malignancies .

Up to 30% of patients with cancer develop cerebral metastasis. Autopsy studies of patients who die of cancer revealed that CNS metastases occur in about 25% of patients. In patients with no history of cancer a cerebral metastasis was the presenting symptom in 15% (EFNS, 2006). Highest incidence of brain metastases is seen in 5th to 7th decade of life.

Metastases most commonly spread via through hematogenous route. The brain parenchyma is the most common site (80%), followed by the skull and dura (15%). Direct extension to brain from a cancer of adjacent structures like cancers of nasopharynx, paranasal sinuses, middle ear (e.g. squamous cell carcinoma, esthenioneuroblastoma) is much less common than hematogenous spread . Diffuse leptomeningeal (pial) and subarachnoid space infiltrations are relatively uncommon, accounting for just 5% of all cases. Brain metastases are preferably located in arterial border zones and at the junction of cerebral cortex and subcortical white matter. Only about 3-5% occur in basal ganglia region. About 15% of metastases are found in the cerebellum. The midbrain, pons and medulla oblongata are uncommon sites and account for less than 1% of metastases. Other rare sites include the choroid plexus, ventricular ependyma, pituitary gland and retinal choroid. The metastasis may also occur through the CSF pathway and may present as drop metastasis. Primary brain tumors like germinoma and medulloblastoma may spread along CSF pathways. Some systemic cancer like lymphomas and leukemias involve leptomeninges and is known as meningeal carcinomatosis. It is a diffuse metastasis in the leptomeninges by carcinomatous infiltration.

Single metastasis accounts for one third to one quarter of patients with brain metastasis. About 20% of patients have two lesions, 30% have three or more and only 5% have more than 5 lesions.

The most common sources of brain metastases in adults are, in descending order, lung cancer (especially small cell and adenocarcinoma), breast cancer, melanoma, renal carcinoma and colon cancer. In children in descending order of frequency, they are leukemia, lymphoma and sarcoma (osteogenic sarcoma, rhabdomyosarcoma and Ewing sarcoma). Melanoma, although constitute only 4% of all cancers, has the highest propensity to result in brain metastasis.

The average period required for the development of brain metastasis from lung cancer is 4 to 10 months, whereas it is approximately 3 years in breast cancer.

Histopathology of the lesion usually reflects the tissue of origin, i.e., the primary site of cancer. The histological features are as diverse as in the primary tumors from which they arise. Metastatic choriocarcinoma should be considered in the differential diagnosis of hemorrhagic intracranial masses in females of child bearing age and surgically resected blood clot should be examined histologically for determining the etiology.

As with other intracranial space occupying lesions the symptoms and signs depend on the size and site of the lesion, raised intracranial pressure, hemorrhage, meningeal irritation and hydrocephalus. Headache, seizures and focal neurologic deficits are the most common presenting symptoms of parenchymal metastases. Detailed neuropsychological testing demonstrates cognitive impairment in 65% of patients with brain metastsasis.

Preoperative metastatic work up includes detailed history and systemic examination to detect the primary cancer, metastases elsewhere in the body and to rule out other diagnosis like brain abscess, tuberculosis, toxoplasmosis, neurocysticercosis, resolving hematoma, lymphoma, hemangioblastoma and glioblastoma.

Chest X-ray, radiograph of the spine, ultrasound of abdomen and pelvis, trans rectal ultrasound, mammography, bronchoscopy, upper GI and lower GI endoscopy, bone marrow examination, radionuclide bone scan, serum electrophoresis, intravenous pyelogram (IVP), CT scan of the brain, chest, abdomen and pelvis, positron emission tomography (PET)-CT or PET-MRI may be required for detection of the systemic cancer. Other important investigations include erythrocyte sedimentation rate (ESR), C- reactive protein (CRP) as markers of infection, Western Blot Test for HIV status, Gram stain, and blood and urine culture to identify hematogenous origin to an abscess. Few investigations are very costly and associated with risks and are required in very rare circumstances.

CT scan and MR are the most commonly used techniques for detecting brain metastases. Brain metastasis appears discrete ring or disc like at subcortical location, at the junction of grey and white matter, with enhancement and extensive surrounding edema which is disproportionate to the size of the lesion. FLAIR image, contrast image, magnetization transfer(MT), MR angiography (MRA), Diffusion weighted imaging (DWI), fat suppression, MR spectroscopy further enhance the value of MRI as the investigation of choice for detecting CNS metastasis.

In carcinomatous meningitis MRI may reveal nodular contrast enhanced lining along the CSF pathways with or without hydrocephalus. FLAIR sequence is of particular value as it may reveal the neoplastic spread along the spinal cord and spinal nerves.

Prominent lipid signal is the dominating peak on MRS in the majority of brain metastases. However, lipid is also common in cellular processes including inflammation and necrosis. Choline is generally elevated, and Cr is depressed or absent in most metastases.

CSF examination may reveal carcinomatous cells. Meningeal biopsy is indicated when imaging fails to support the diagnosis but this disease is strongly suspected.

About 11% patients with known primary cancer do not have metastatic lesion, despite the fact that CT scan or MRI suggest so. Half of these patients can have potentially curable inflammatory and so a histopathological confirmation must be obtained before planning treatment.

Whole body PET-CT scanner can detect any significant residual or recurrent FDG avid lesion at the primary cancer site, or status of the lymph nodes, lungs, liver, spleen, kidneys, urinary bladder and other organs and systems like skeletal system. PET is used to evaluate the therapy response and to assess the disease status. However, PET does not distinguish secondary from primary neoplasms and may be false positive in some benign lesions of the brain.

Therapeutic approaches include steroid therapy, stereotactic biopsy, neurosurgical resection, brachytherapy, SRS, WBRT, chemotherapy and combinations of treatment. Patient selection for a particular type of treatment is paramount in order to maximize survival and neurologic function whilst avoiding unnecessary treatment. Clinical and radiographic prognostic factors and histology of the lesion are the most important determinants of the outcome. Good prognostic indicators include Karnofsky performance status (KPS) of more than 70, age less than 65 and controlled primary tumor and no extracranial metastasis. Other prognostic factors include the sensitivity of the tumor to therapy and number and location of CNS metastases.

Anti edema measures like Frusemide, Mannitol , Glycerol, Acetazolamide and Dexamethasone reduce the raised ICP. Steroids have an oncolytic effect and cause shrinkage of metastatic lymphomas. The mainstay of treatment for brain metastsasis over the past 5 decades has been corticosteroids and WBRT. Non randomized studies suggest that WBRT increases the median survival time by 3-4 months over approximately 1 month without treatment and 2 months with corticosteroids.

Radiotherapy can be delivered by fractionated external beam irradiation, small field streotactic irradiation (stereotactic radiotherapy) or interstitial implantation (brachytherapy) (Dagnew et al, 2007, Patchell et al 1998) . For whole brain radiation therapy (WBRT), the most common regimen employed is 35 Gy delivered in 2.5 Gy fractions over 14 treatment days. Daily fraction of more than 3 Gy likely increases the risk of neurotoxicity.

Stereotactic radiotherapy (SRT) is delivered using a linear accelerator. A fractionated schedule is followed maintaining the targeting technique of SRS.

For neoplastic spread to the spinal cord, treatment involves the irradiation of the entire neuraxis with chemotherapy including methotrxate, cytosine arabinoside, and thiotepa. Intra-CSF drug therapy can also also be given. Topotecan, an inhibitor of totpisomerase-1, crosses the blood brain barrier (BBB) and may be effective in treatment of brain metastasis from small cell lung and breast cancer. Temozolamide, an oral alkylating agent also crosses BBB is useful in treating brain metastasis.

Stereotactic radiosurgery (SRS) is a relatively recent therapeutic option that has significantly improved the effectiveness of and morbidity associated with radiation therapy. SRS may use gamma knife (GK) or linear accelerator (LINAC, CyberKnife) delivers a single large dose of focused radiation to lesions localized by stereotaxy. SRS is useful for lesions less than 3 cm to 4 cm where a radiation of 1,600 – 3,500 cGy is delivered in a single sitting. A major advantage of this technique over conventional surgery is that it can treat surgically inaccessible tumors in the eloquent area of the brain. SRS is a safe alternative to surgical excision in elderly frail patients with associated medical conditions, such as diabetes mellitus, hypertension. SRS is a non invasive procedure and it obviates the need of multiple craniotomies in a patient with multiple metastases. Some tumors are very sensitive to radiation like metastasis from lymphoma, germ cell tumor and small cell lung cancer where SRS is the treatment of choice.

Surgical resection is the treatment of choice in all the patients where lesion is surgically accessible, associated with significant mass effect and hydrocephalus. If the lesion is more than 4 cm in size, or highly cystic then surgical intervention is definitely better than SRS. If a patient presents with mass effect, local irritation of the adjoining brain tissue, raised intracranial pressure and tumor is in surgically accessible area of the brain then immediate tumor excision or decompression should be done. If the primary cancer is controlled and the life expectancy is more than 3 months, the surgery is indicated. Surgery is life saving and helps in establishing the histopathological diagnosis. The importance of diagnosis is paramount when the diagnosis of brain metastasis is in question. This is important because as many as

10%-15% of patients with a clinical diagnosis of metastasis may actually have non metastatic lesions such as abscess.

Surgical excision should be considered for patients with good KPS score, minimal or no evidence of extracranial disease and surgically accessible brain metastasis. Surgery is needed in cancers which are resistant to radiation like thyroid carcinoma, renal cell carcinoma and melanoma. A certain, immediate and predictable outcome of surgical resection and long term local control metastatic lesion are major advantages over radiation based treatment modalities.

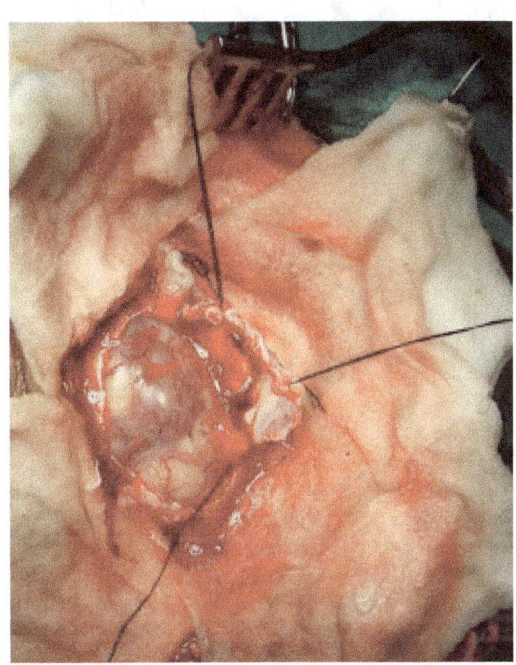

Intraoperative photograph of a frontal lobe metastasis

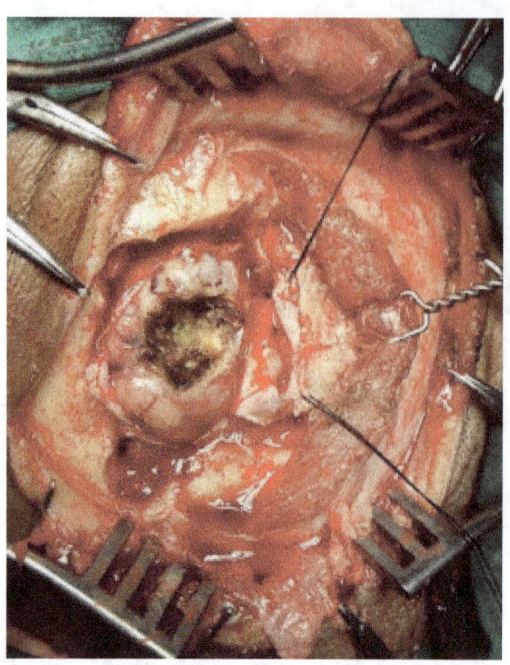

Intraoperative photograph showing frontal lobe after excision of metastasis

Stereotactic biopsy should be an option for lesions located in inaccessible and eloquent area of the brain.

After surgery or stereotactic radiosurgery (SRS), adjuvant whole brain radiation therapy (WBRT) is recommended. It is an effort to erradicate residual cancer cells at the resected site and to eliminate microscopic foci at distant sites within the brain, thereby, reducing the risk of tumor recurrence.

Long term follow up of the patient is mandatory for evaluation of neurological status, complications of chemoradiation therapy, detection of recurrence or appearance of any new lesion, neuro-cognitive impairment and for neuro-rehabilitation and supportive care.

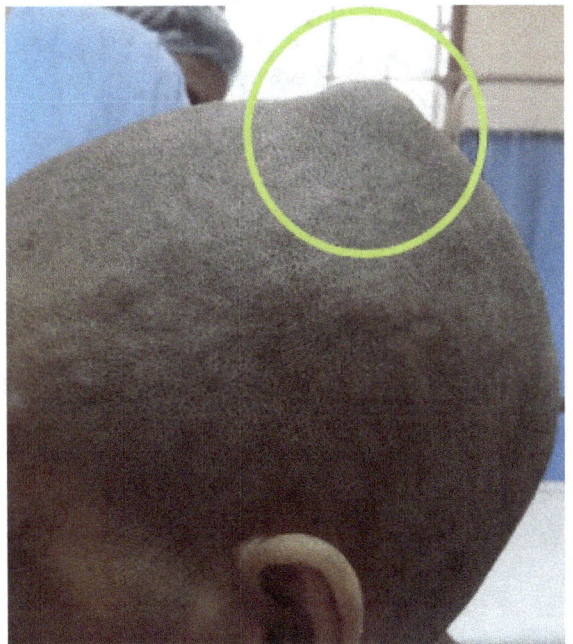

A middle age female patient had presented with swelling in the head and history of seizures

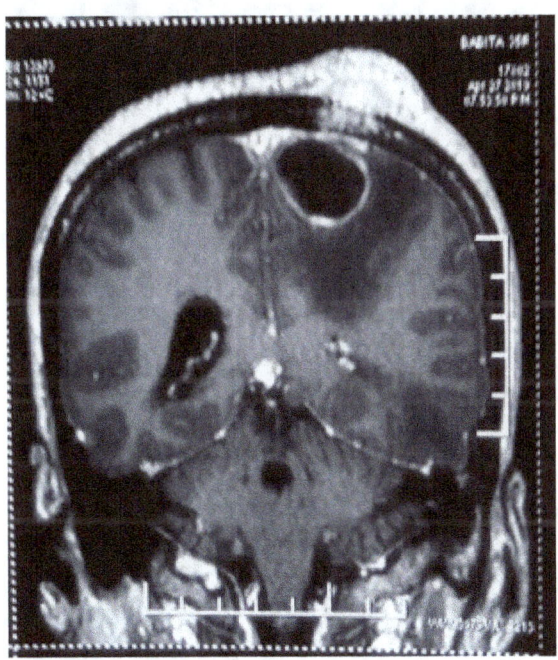

MRI of brain the above mentioned patient showing scalp swelling and involvement of the cranium and intracranial cystic lesion with enhancement

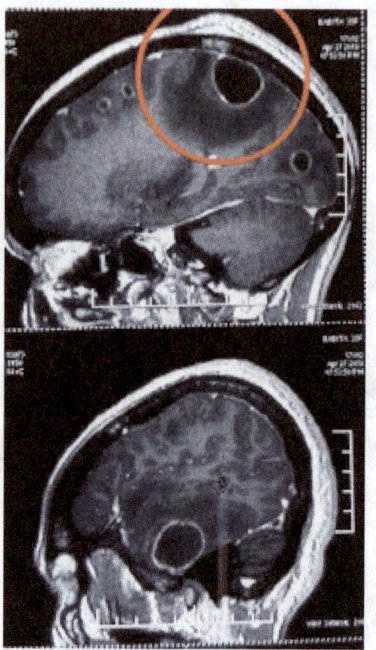

This middle aged female had multiple intracranial metastses without detectable systemic primary cancer.

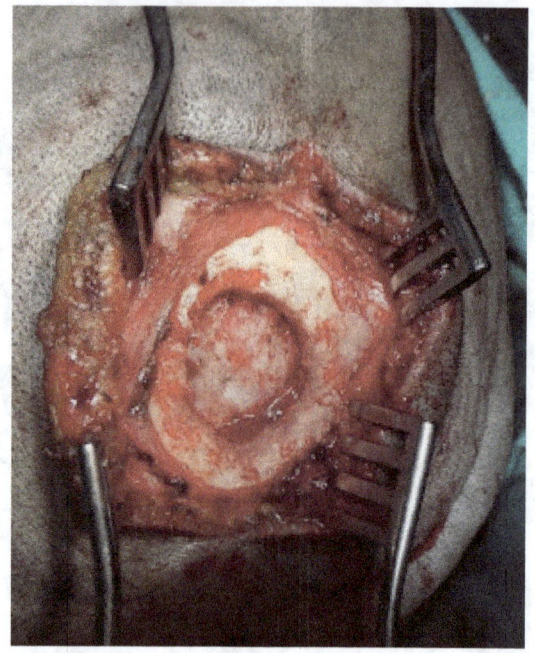

Intraoperative image shows defect in the cranial bone as seen after excision of the soft to firm swelling just beneath the scalp incision. Tumor was adherent to dura also. Intracranial lesion was mainly cystic with soft, suckable and moderately vascular surrounding solid compnent of the metastatic lesion.

Conclusion

In a suspected case of brain metastasis choice of investigation, neuro-imaging and therapy must be decided by the treating team based on a firm understanding of the prognostic indicators and other parameters. Patient selection is the cornerstone of management with brain metastasis. Prompt decision and aggressive management with combined modality of treatment minimizes cost of care, maximizes the clinical outcome and reduces the mortality and morbidity of patients with brain metastases.

References

[1] Mark S. Greenberg, *Handbook of neurosurgery*, 7th edition, Thieme (2010), pp 702-710, ISBN 978-1-60406-326-4.

[2] Chapter : Metastatic Brain tumors, Ramamurthy R, Harinivas in Ramamurthy & Tandon's *Manual of Neurosurgery*, P.N.Tandon, Ravi Ramamurthy, Pradeep Kumar Jain N., First Edition, ISBN 978-93-5152-192-1(2014) pp 1049-1064.

[3] Anne G. Osborn. *Osborn Brain imaging, pathology and anatomy.*, 2nd edition (Amirsys)

[4] Eichler A.F., and Loeffler J.S. Multidisciplinary management of brain metastases. *The Oncologist*, 2007; 12: 884-898.

[5] Mintz, A.; J.Perry, K. Spinthoff, A. Chambers and N.Laperriere. Management of single brain metastasis: a practice guideline. *Current Oncology,* Volume 14, number 4,130-143.

[6]. WHO Classification of tumors of the central nervous system, Edited by D.N.Louis, H.Olgaki, O.D. Weistler, and W. K. Cavenee. Chapter: Metastatic tumors of the CNS by P. Wesseling, A.V. Deimling, K.D. Aldap.

[7]. EFNSguidelines on diagnosis and treatment of brain metastasis: report of an EFNS task force. *European journal of Neurology*, 2006, 13; 674-681.

[8] H.R. Winn, *Youmans Neurological Surgery*, 6th Edition, Vol 2 (Elsevier Saunders) Chapter: Metastatic brain tumors. By F.F.Lang, E.L.Chang, D.Suki, D.M. Wildrick, R. Sawaya.

[9] Ramamurthy, K. Sridhar, M.C.Vasudevan. *Textbook of operative neurosurgery*, Ed Vol.1, B.I. Publication Pvt Ltd, New Delhi. Chapter: Surgical management of brain metastasis, By V.K.Khosla, B.S.Sharma.

[10] Alexander Chi, Ritsuko Komaki. Treatment of brain metastasis from lung cancer, *Cancer* 2010, 2,2100-2137.

[11] Andrew D. Norden, Patrick Y. Wen and Santosh Kesari. Brain metastases. *Current Opinion in Neurology*, 2005, 18;654-661.

[12] Remi Nader, Abdulrahman J. Sabbagh, Thieme. Neurosurgery Case review Questions and Answers ,.Chapter, Case 17 : single brain metastases Joseph A. Shehadi and Brian Seaman, Chapter, Case 18: Multiple brain metastases. Ramez Malak and Robert Moumdijian.

[13] Timothy Siu, Frederick F. Lang. Surgical management of cerebral metastasis. Page 178-91.Chapter in Textbook : *Schmidek & Sweet operative Neurosurgical techniques, indications, methods and results,* Alfredo Quinones- Hinojosa, 6th edition, (Elsevier Saunders).

[14] Gaspar L, Scott C, Rotman M, et al. Recursive partitioning analysis (RPA) of prognostic factors in three Radiation Therapy Oncology Group (RTOG) brain metastases trials . *International Journal of Radiation Oncology, Biology, Physics* 1997; 37: 745-751.

[15] Wong ET, Berkenbit A. The role of topotecan in the treatment of brain metastasis. *Oncologist*, 2004; 9:68-79.

[16] Dagnew E, Kanski J, Mc Dermott MW, et al. Management of newly diagnosed single brain metastasis using resection and permanent iodine-125 seeds without initial whole-brain radiotherapy: a two institution experience. NeurosurgFocus 2007; 22(3):E3

[17] Patchell RA, Tibbs PA, Regine WF, et al. Postoperative radiotherapy on the treatment of single metastasis to the brain: a randomized trial JAMA 1998; 280: 1485-1489.

STROKE

The term "Heart attack" is very common used term and well understood by common people for a condition in which heart is affected and patient requires urgent medical treatmnt. Similarly in stroke, blood supply to the brain is affected and patient requires urgent medical attention.

The brain is critically dependent on an uninterrupted supply of oxygenated blood. About 18% of the total blood volume in body circulates in the brain, which accounts for about 2% of body weight. Loss of consciousness occurs in less than 15 seconds after blood flow to the brain has stopped, and irreparable damage to the brain tissue occurs within 5 minutes.

Cerebrovascular accident or cerebrovascular disease or stroke occurs as a result of vascular compromise or hemorrhage and is one of the most frequent sources of neurologic disability.

Abrupt onset of Neurologic deficit is caused by inadequate perfusion of a region of brain.

Stroke is a common cause of neurological disability and death in elderly persons. Arterial thrombosis with occlusion of the cerebral arteries is the most common cause of stroke.

Most common modifiable risk factors are hypertension, cigarette smoking, obesity, increased blood lipids, heavy alcohol consumption, poor control of diabetes mellitus, stress, etc.

TIA (Transient ischemic attack)

Episode of focal neurological dysfunction as a result of ischemia which resolves completely within 24 hours.

TIA are important determinant of stroke. around 30-50% of cases had previous transient ischemic attacks.

STROKE or CVA

About 85% of strokes are Ischemic and 15% Hemorrhagic.

HEMORRHAGIC STROKE

About 20% of strokes are hemorrhagic which is due to the spontaneous intracerebral hematoma (ICH). Hemorrhage most commonly results from rupture of the small penetrating arteries damaged by the degenerative effects of chronic hypertension.. In 1868, Charcot and Bouchard described the rupture of " microaneurysms" as the cause of ICH.

Common cause of spontaneous intracerbral hematoma in elderly is hypertensive bleed. As commonly seen in elderly that there is unnoticed hypertension in many elderly persons who are not aware about this condition or on irregular treatment of hypertension. Common site of hypertensive bleed is basal ganglia.

So, the commonest cause of spontaneous intracerebral hematoma in adults is a hypertensive arteriosclerotic basal ganglionic bleed. The median age of spontaneous intracerebral hemorrhage is about 56 years. The common clinical features are sudden onset severe headache, vomiting, slurring of speeh, depressed level of consciousness and weakness of face and limbs.

Commonest cause is long standing hypertension, irregular antihypertensive medication, history of smoking and alcohol intake, diabetes and lack of physical exercise.

CT scan of brain is the initial investigation.

LOWER BACKACHE

Lower back pain is a very common complaint in all age groups. We all have experienced back pain at some time in our life time. Sometimes, it persists and affects our routine and becomes a matter of concern. But, in fact, most of the times it is just stiffness or muscle strain due to hard work, prolong standing, sternuous excercise, play, or after lifting some heavy object. Such back pain is not due to any underlying disease. Mild or moderate level of pain gets relieved by taking analgesics (like an adult may take Diclofenac 50 mg after meal, SOS) and after taking rest. The other causes of backache are muscle sprain, muscle pull, strain, wrong posture, etc.
Pain is a subjective sensation and the complaint of backache may vary from person to person. For example, for an athlete the lower backache after a prolong run or play may not be of a great concern but similar intensity of pain may be very debilitating for an old age person.

So, mild back pain which can be explained on the basis of obvious cause like prolong walk and play should not be investigated. Bed rest is the best medical advice for relieving backache.

However, severe persistent backache without any obvious precipitating factor may warrant a consultation with the medical specialist. Orthopedicians, Physiotherapists, Sport medicine physicians, Neurologists and Neurosurgeons commonly encounter patients with complaints of lower backache.

One of the common causes of lower backache is lumbar spondylosis, which is a progressive degenerative disease of the spine. With aging the water content in the intervertebral disc, ligament and bone is gradually decreased and it restricts the movement of the spine. The vertebral column or spine consists of cervical, thoracic, lumbar and sacral part.

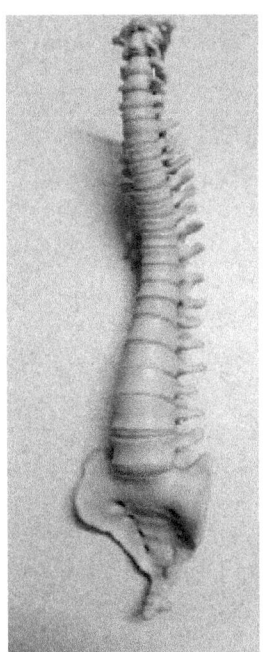

A model image of the entire spine

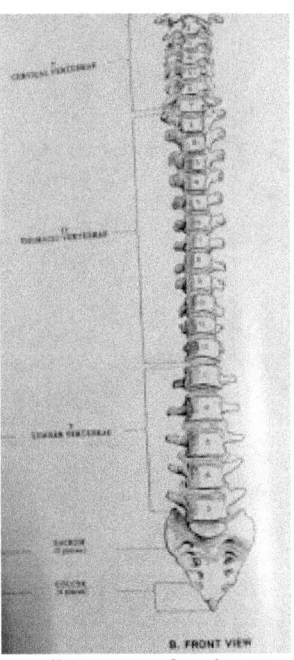

diagram of spine

Cervical part is located on the back of the neck and is the most mobile part. Even without our notice we move our neck and cervical spine for about 80,000 times in a day. So, the cervical spine is very prone for the degenerative changes in older age group. Because thoracic spine (chest) is relatively less mobile due to rib cage it is less prone for spondylosis. Lumbar is the lower part and it bears the weight of the body. Due to excessive weight bearing this part of spine is prone for slip disc or listhesis.

What is Lumbar Spondylosis or Lumbar Degenerative disease?

Lumbar Spondylosis is medical term to describe a degenerative disease of the lower part of vertebral column. Our vertebral column or back bone or spine consists of four areas, namely: cervical, thoracic, lumbar and sacral region. Lower part of the spine, i.e, region below the rib cage, consists of lumar and sacral region. There are 5 lumbar vertebrae with intervertebral discs between two adjacent vertebral bodies.So, progressive wear and tear of this region may cause different types of diseaes. Lumbar spondylosis may lead to lumbar canal stenosis, prolapse of intervertebral disc (PIVD) and spondylolisthesis. Lumbar spondylosis is a common cause of lower backache.

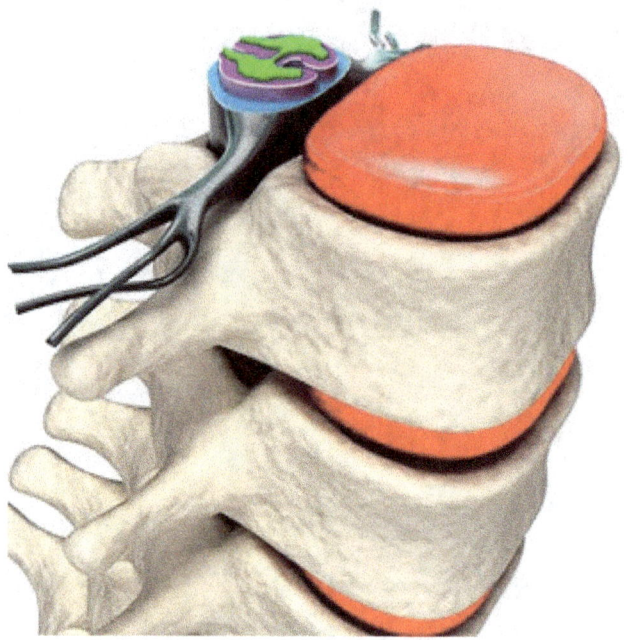

Image showing parts of the vertebral bodies with disc. Spinal cord is contained inside the spinal column which is formed anteriorly by the vertebral bodies and discs and bounded posteriorly by the lamina and spinous processes. In this image spinal nerve roots are seen emerging from the spinal cord (source: http://www.medicinenet.com)

Our vertebral column consists of vertebrae and the intervertebral disc which are strengthened by many ligaments. The vertebral column contains vertebral canal within this bony canal a 45 centimetre long spinal cord is contained. The spinal nerves come out through the intervertebral foramina which are bordered by disc, pedicle, vertebral body and facet joints. So, any abnormality of disc, facet joint or vertebral joint leads to narrowing of the intervertebral neural foramina which compress the spinal nerves causing pain and later neurological deficit in the form of loss of sensation and muscle weakness.

What causes Lumbar Spondylosis?

It is due to increased stress over the lumbar vertebrae which causes protrusion of the intervertebral disc, calcification of the ligaments and osteoplytes formation . Osteophytes are the abnormal bony projections. Stress over the vertebrae is mostly due to increased body weight, sedentary lifestyle, wrong posture or due to old age. Due to many risk factors, the disc may age prematurely and dries up (disc dessication), leading to narrowing of the disc space. This in turn decreases the flexibility of the spine and osteophyte formation in the vertebral bodies. Nerve compression causes nerve edema, alteration in nutritional transport along the nerve, and local inflammation, therefore bed rest and anti-inflammatory medications may relieve the symptoms of the patient.

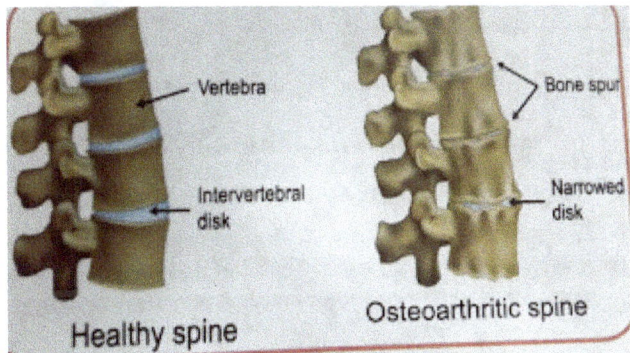

Image showing a normal part of spine and part of osteoarthritic spine

What are the common symptoms of Lumbar Spondylosis?

Lumbar canal stenosis is commonly a disease of the old age and commonly occurs due to hypertrophy of the ligamentum flavum. Patient complains of pain in lower back (Claudication) after walking for a long distance (Claudication distance). Gradually , over a time , this distance decreases and person starts complaining of lower backache even after walking for 100 meters. Pain gets relieved on taking rest or in sitting position. There is no pain on bending. I this way pain due to Lumbar canal stenosis differs from the pain caused by PIVD. Pain due to disc prolapse usually increases on bending.

This problem is very commonly seen in old age persons. Initially they are able to walk for a long distance with very mild pain at the end of the walk. But, gradually with advancing age the intensity of pain increases and they start feeling pain even after walking for 200 meters or so. The moment they take rest and sit idle for a moment pain subsides. So, sitting is not painful. Some people find no difficulty in cycling but prolong walking induces lower backache.

PIVD

Prolapse of the intervertebral disc or PIVD is a very common neurosurgical condition. **Prolapse** or buldge or protrusion of the intervertebral disc causes compression of the spinal nerve which causes lower backache. PIVD causes pain in the legs and sometimes bladder & bowel symptoms. Pain in the lower back is usually caused by muscle strain. It may also include sciatica (pain that radiates from the back to the buttock and down into the leg). Onset of pain may be immediate or occur some hours after an activity.

Pain and stiffness may be ongoing, or only occur when you are in certain positions. The pain may get worse by coughing, sneezing, bending, or twisting. Even sitting may induce pain. Such type of lower backache only lying on bed in certain posture may relief pain.

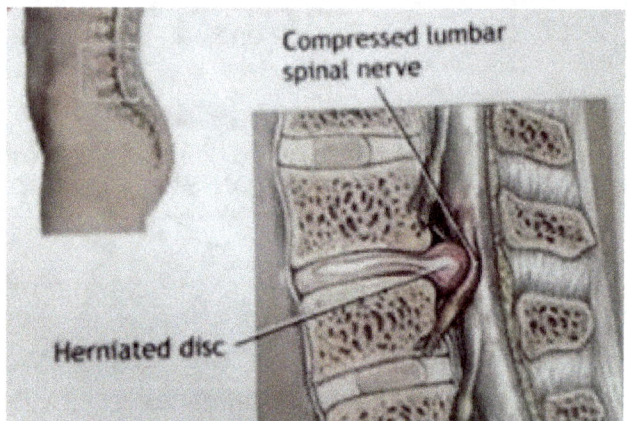

Image showing prolapse of the intervertebral disc posteriorly causing compression of the spinal nerve

Spondylolisthesis is another type of degeneration. The one vertebral body is slipped over the another vertebral body. It also leads to pain in lower back.

Spondylolisthesis is very common in lumbosacral region of the spine. L4 vertebra is displaced over the L5 vertebra (L4/L5 spondylolisthesis) or L5 is displaced over the S1 verterbra (L5/S1 spondylolisthesis). In old aged females osteoporosis is very common and the ligaments are also weakened , so the degenerative spondylolisthesis is very common in lumbosacral region.

How to recognize Lumbar Spondylosis?

One should not ignore the severe lower backache and particularly if pain is radiating to lower limb or associated with numbness or weakness of the lower limb. Investigations like X-ray of the lumbosacral spine and MRI scan of the lower back can diagnose this problem.

Sometimes, X-ray of the spine in standing posture with bending forward & backword is required to diagnose spondylolisthesis.

MRI of the lumbosacral spine is the preferred investigation for diagnosis of cause of lower backache. It will show the alignment of the lumbar vertebrae and intervertebral disc, dural sac, lumbar canal diameter and nerve roots. So, even a minimal disc bulge is visible on MRI. MRI may exclude other causes of the lower backache line nerve sheath tumors, any other disease of this region like Potts spine (tuberculosis), Multiple Myeloma, etc.

So, Plain X-ray and MRI of the spine are indispensable for the diagnosis of any disease of the spine. Sometimes, CT scan of the spine may be required.

What are the treatment options?

Almost everyone experiences pain after exercise or after a prolong walk or on exertion. So, all cases of mild lower backache need not to be investigated.

Treatment will depend on the cause of the pain. Usually a strict bed rest, lumbosacral belt and analgesics (mild pain drugs such as aspirin, ibuprofen, or acetaminophen) for a short period of time can relieve the symptoms.

Many treatment options are available. Physiotherapy measures like short wave diathermy, ultrasound therapy , traction and exercise therapy may help in chronic cases of lumbar spondylosis.

Sometimes stronger pain relieving drugs, muscle relaxants, and drugs to reduce inflammation may be needed.

Urgent neurosurgical intervention is required if there is high degree of degeneration of veretebrae, or if a disk is protruded,or associated canal stenosis or weakness or decreased sensation in the lower limbs or difficulty in urination. Neurosurgical Microscopic discoictomy, endoscopic discoidectomy are common surgical interventions.

In some cases, like severe spondylolisthesis, spinal surgical fixation with implants is required.

Can lumbar spondylosis be prevented?

Primary prevention of lumbar spondylosis is possible by regular exercise, physiotherapy, correct posture and weight reduction. Once diagnosed with lumbar spondylosis a patient should avoid lifting heavy weight & bending forward.

Posture correction, use of correct lifting techniques, avoidance of sudden twisting movement of back, use of cushion at lower back to maintain lumbar lordotic curve is mandatory to prevent progressive degeneration of lumbar spine.

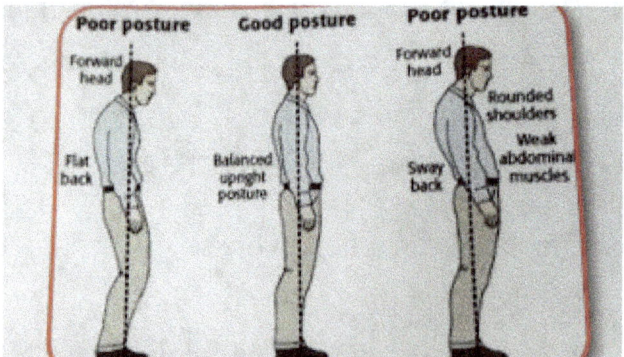

Image suggests correct standing posture standing posture without a hunch or lordosis

Surgery prevents further deterioration is severe cases. Discoidectomy and Spinal fixation may treat severe cases of spondylolisthesis and prevent further neurological deficit. Severe cases of disc extrusion should be operated to avoid foot drop and cauda equina syndrome.

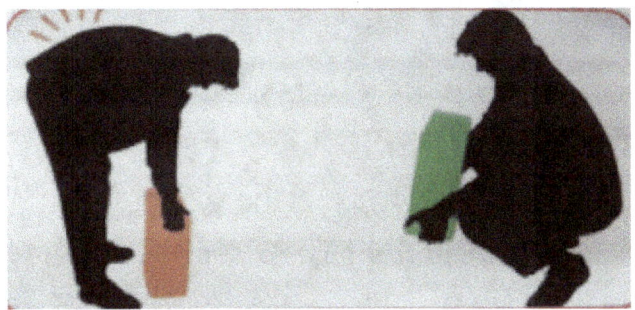

Lifting of the heavy object in stooping posture is common cause of acute disc prolapse. In first image a person is lifting object in stooping posture which makes him prone to the acute neurological deficit due to PIVD. In second part the person is trying to lift the object not in stooping posture and it may be relatively safe.

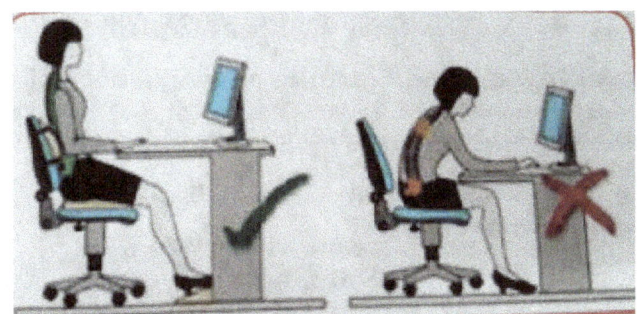

Working over computer table for a long period in incorrect posture leads to early onset of spondylosis

What are the Rehabilitation options for patients with lumbar spondylosis?

Neurological rehabilitation is a therapeutic program designed to improve function. Various rehabilitative measure like Isometric back exercise, core stability exercises and mobilization of lower limb joints and stretching of tight muscles are done to maintain normal anatomical integrity of the spine. Different interventions like Ultrasonic therapy, Transcutaneous Electrical Nerve Stimulation (TENS) , Short Wave Diathermy ,Traction and Interferential Therapy are available for rehabilitation of the lumbar spondylosis patients.

In case of severe neurological deficit rehabilitative therapy is available to promote compensatory strategies to attain maximum possible functional independence. These measures are mainly motor retraining, Neurodevelopmental therapy (NDT) , ADL training , Assistive and adaptive techniques and ergonomic rehabilitation.

Other causes of lower backache like Sponylolisthesis

SPINAL TRAUMA

OSTEOPOROSIS

NERVE SHEATH TUMORS, infections of the vertebrae like spinal tuberculosis,

OSTEOARTHRITIS OF HIP JOINT

Should also be investigated.

X-ray of the lumbosacral spine (anteroposterior and lateral view may provide an initial clue to the diagnosis.

For diagnosis of L1 vertebra collapse fracture, x- ray film of dorsolumbar spine is advised. This is very common fracture in people who fall from height.

MRI is the investigation of choice. It shows intervertebral disc, ligaments, vertebral bodies, integrity of the spinal cord.

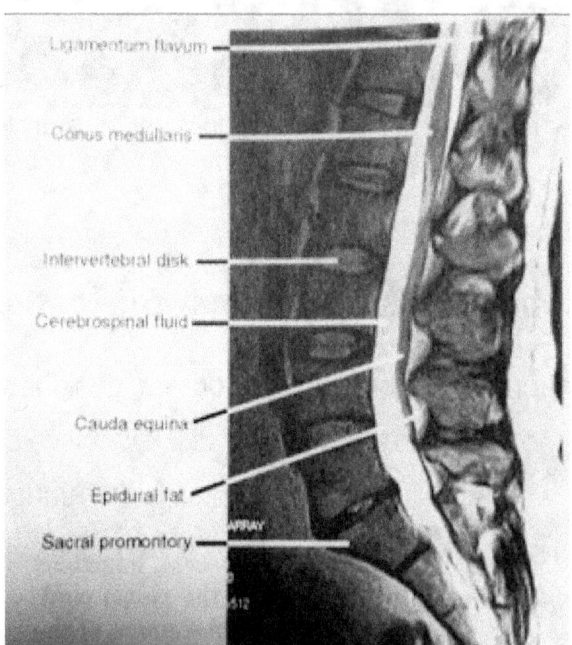

Labelled diagram of MRI side (sagittal view) showing different parts of lumbosacral region of spine

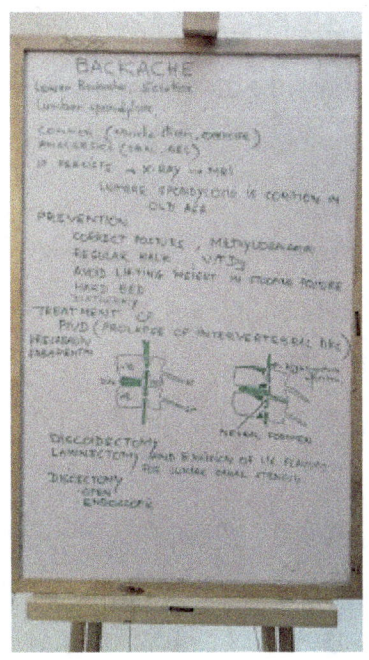

Sources
Naturopathy & yogic management of Lumbar spondylosis . Booklet of Central council for research in yoga and naturopathy (An autonomous organisation under Ministry of AYUSH , Govt of India), and online resources

EPILEPSY (SEIZURES, FITS, CONVULSIONS)

Epilepsy is a symptom which indicates that there is some problem in the physiology of brain.

So, if a person presents with seizures a detailed work up should be done. It begins with detailed history.

Broadly epilepsy is classified as:

GTCS: Generalized Tonic Clonic Seizures

CPS: Complex Partial sezures (Usually due to temporal lobe involvement, may be associated with hallucinations or other complex symptoms)

Focal seizures

Focal seizures with secondary generalization

In infants and children of less than five year of age, if single episode of seizure occurs during high grade fever, it is most likely a Febrile convulsion for which long term antileptic medication is not required.

In majority of cases, the cause of the seizure is not known. When neuroradiology does not reveal any abnormality and other causes are ruled out after detailed work up, it is labeled as idiopathic epilepsy.

The common causes are infections, neoplasm, trauma, vascular lesions, development, etc. The **infective** granulomas (Tubercular, Neurocysticercus, Toxoplasma), Abscess, Meningitis, encephalitis are the common infective etiologies. Head injury (Extradural hematoma, Subdural hematoma, Diffuse axonal injury, etc) may present as **Post traumatic Epilepsy**, immediately following trauma or at later stage, known as Post Traumatic Late onset Epilepsy.

Brain tumors can present as seizures. All the tumors which involve or compress the cerebral hemispheres may present with seizures.

Supratentorial **Gliomas** and **Meningiomas** have very high incidence of seizures. Although, Meningioma is an extra axial lesion as it arises from dura (originates from Arachnoidal Cap Cells), it is associated with brain edema, and so presents with seizures.

Brain metastasis is also associated with brain edema and presents with seizures.
Arterivenous malformation in the cerebral hemispheres usullay presents with seizures in children. **Subarachnoid hemorrhage** due to rupture of the intracranial aneurysm may present with seizures.

Other brain abnormalities like Schizencephaly, arachnoid cyst, **epidermoid** may present with seizures.

Mesial Temporal Sclerosis usually presents with Complex partial seizures.

How to investigate a case of Epilepsy?

History, Physical Examination may reveal a clue to the diagnosis, like Tuberculosis, Primary cancers elsewhere in the body.

CT scan or MRI of the brain with contrast with MR spectroscopy

EEG

How to treat Epilepsy?

Sodium **Valproate** or **Phenyton** should be used as primary antiepileptic medication, because these two antiepiletics had been in clinical use since very long time, their complications are well known and very much predictable. In case of status epilepticus, their injectable forms are available so a loading dose can easily be delivered. Because of injectable, neurosurgeons can also use them during perioperative period.

Carbamazepine can aso be used as primary antiepileptic medication.

It is very easy to remember the doses of these three very commonly used drugs.

Phenyton, 5 mg/ kg body weight (so, in an adult of about 50 kg weight give Phenytoin 100 mg TthreeTimes a Day)

Carbamazepine, 10mg/ kg body weight (so, in an adult of about 50 kg weight give CBZ 200 mg TDS)

Valproate, 15 mg/ kg body weight (so, in an adult of about 50 kg weight give Valproate 300 mg TDS).Valproate is a very common conditions, like Migraine, Mood disorders, so it may help in comorbid conditions,as well)

Seizures are usually controlled with single antiepileptic drug if prescribed in proper dosage. If it is not controlled increase the dose.

For Long term Antiepileptic medication :Another add on therapy should only be given when the maximum dose of the first drug is already in use and seizures are still uncontrolled.

The first drug to be added is usually Clobazam.

For example, If in an adult operated patient of glioma , seizures were controlled earlier with Tab Phenytoin 100mg TDS, if Seizures occur, add 100 mg : So it will be 100 mg 4 times a day, and seizures are not controlled , an addition of Tablet Clobazam 10 mg can control the epilepsy.

Now, another epileptic is vigorously marketed as primary antiepileptic and also as add-on therapy, i.e., Levetiracetam. This drug has also been use in clinical practice with good safety profile. Moreover, the availability of injectable forms are added advantage, for treating status epilepticus.

Many other antiepileptics are used depending upon condition of the patient.

Topiramate is used in cases of migraine and seizure patients with obesity.

NEUROSURGICAL ICU

The resident doctors should know the management of a patient on ventilator. The rationale use antibiotics, dressing, pulse ,BP monitoring, examination of the respiratory system, and interpretation of the chest X-ray and change of the ventilator setting are the important skills for the resident doctors.

Respiratory System, Pneumonia, Chronic Pulmoary Obstructive Disease (COPD)- Emphysema, Chronic Brochitis, Brochiectasis, Asthtma, Carcinoma of lung

Respiratory system is very important in clinical setting. Every doctor must be aware about this system. As oxygen is important for life, similarly understanding of the respiratory system is essential for sustaining the medical practice of any doctor. Good aspect of this fact is that anybody can learn the entire respiratory system in a very simple way and theory of the respiratory system can be understood in one page and its usual practice in clinical setting makes every doctor confident in understanding of the respiratory system.

Common symptoms of diseases of the respiratory system are dyspnea, cough, fever, hemoptysis, chest pain, weight loss. So, just knowing the details about each symptom can help in making a provisional diagnosis of diseases of the respiratory system.

History-

Dyspnea or Dyspnoea is difficulty in breathing which may be in the form of breathlessness.

Cough may be dry of with sputum (Expectoration).

Dry cough is commonly seen in Legionella.

Purulent Sputum- Klebsiella (Thick Red Currant Jelly like sputum)

So, the history taking is important in making a diagnosis of respiratory system. History of tubercular contact is common in Tuberculosis. History of smoking is common in COPD and lung carcinoma. History of significant weight loss is common in Tuberculosis and lung carcinoma.

Clinical Examination of patients should be done in a systematic manner. Start with

Inspection-

On inspection alone certain diagnosis of respiratory system can be made. Measure respiratory rate, observe the pattern of the breathing (abdominothoracic or thoracoabdominal), Dyspnea, use of accessory muscles of respiration, movement of the chest, any structural abnormality of the chest wall, curvature of the spine (kyphosis, scoliosis), any tumor of the chest, e.g., chondroma.

Palpation-

Extent of chest expansion can be measured by placing both palm across the spine and asking the patient to take deep breath.

On palpation of the chest wall cutaneous emhysema can be detected. Cutaneous emphysema is the air in the subcutaneous tissue of the chest and it feels like crepitations while compressing skin over the chest wall.

Vocal fremitus is examined by placing the ulnar aspect of the hand over different areas of the chest wall feeling the vibration of the sound with and while patients produces repetitive words like one, one , one. Vocal fremitus is decreased in pleural effusion but it is increased in pneumonia.

Extent of any bony tumor like chondroma of the ribs or costochondral junction can be felt by palpation.

Fracture of the ribs can be detected on palpation. Tenderness of the chest wall can be detected on palpation. Any paraspinal collection or cold abscess can also be detected on palpation which is very common in Tuberculosis.

Percussion-

Placing the middle finger of of one hand over the chest wall and tapping with index finger of other hand will commonly elicit tympanic or dull percussion over the chest wall. The normal percussion sound over the lungs is tympanic. In hemothorax the percussion will be dull. In hydropneuomathorax it will dull below and tympanic in upper part of pneumothorax. In Pneumonia (Consolidation of the lungs) it is dull but this is stony dull in case of pleural effusion. Tympanic sound is increased in case of emphysema of the lungs. In pneumothorax the percussion is hyperresonant.

Auscultation-

Auscultation is done with stethoscope and all doctors should own a stethoscope. The usual breath sound are either vesicular or amphoric. The breath sounds are inreased in consolidation ,i.e., in pneumonia. The breath sounds are decreased, i.e., muffled, in pleural effusion. Breath sounds will be decreased in hemothorax.

Crepts are heard in lung infection, pulmonary edema.

Ronchi or whistle like sounds are heard in bronchoconstriction and in asthma.

So, the with clinical examination will be sufficient to make the diagnosis of tension pneumothorax.

Pleural effusion, pneumothorax, hydropneumothorax, pneumonia, emphysema can be provisionally diagnosed on clinical examination itself. It can further be clearly diagnosed with chest X ray.

Investigations-

Chest X-Ray Postero-anterior view (PA) is very common radiological investigation. It helps in diagnosis of rib fracture, flail chest, pneumothorax, hydropneumothorax, COPD, brochiectasis, pleural effusion, Cor pulmonale, cardiomegaly, mediastinal widening, carcinoma lung, Tuberculosis, chest metastasis.

In Pnumonia, cosolidation or cavitation is seen on chest x-ray depending upon type of pneumonia

- In consolidation, the lungs shadow appear radiopaque on chest x ray.
    - Lobar consolidation is seen in pneumococcal pneumonia.
    - Bibasal consolidation is seen in Legionella pneumonia.
    - Patchy shadows- Chlamydia psittaci. If Bilateral then Mycoplasma.
- In cavitation, pneumonia is due to
    - Bilateral cavitation- Staphylococcal
    - Upper lobe cavitation- Klebsiella

Bilateral perihilar interstitial shadowing is seen in Pneumocystis carnii pneumonia.

Tram line and ring shadows are seen in brochiectasis.

Spirometry can diagnose the restrictive and obstructive disease of the lungs.

FEV1 is helpful in the diagnosis of asthma.

V/Q scan (Ventilation perfusion scan)

CT scan or HRCT (High resolution CT scan) of the chest helps in the diagnosis of brochiectasis, and lung carcinoma.

Pulmonary angiography- clot in the 5th order pulmonary artery can be seen in Pulmoary embolism which usually occurs on 10th post operative day.

Bronchoscopy and biopsy

Montoux test, sputum culture and sensitivity test is useful in diagnosis of Tuberculosis.

Legionella serology

Treatment of respiratory diseases

Tension pneumothorax- Tension pneumothorax is a medical emergency. Tracheal deviation is noticed in a patient who complaints of sudden shortness of breaths and neck veins are distended. Patient becomes cyanosed. So, needle thoracocentesis is done immediately.

Pneumororax : oxygen, needle aspiration, chest tube drain.

Hemothorax- chest tube drainage

Bronchogenic carcinoma- It can present with fever if there is secondary pneumonia and it requires antibiotic therapy. Surgery is for Non small cell lung cancer. Radiotherapy is treatment of choice if patient's age is more than 65 years.

Bronchiectasis- steroid inhaler, antibiotics if there is associated infection. Postural drainage.

Pneumonia-

    Streptococcus pneumoniae- Ampicillin or cefuroxime

    Legionella- Erythromycin

    Staphylococcus- Flucloxacillin

    Pneumocystis carnii pneumonia- high dose co-trimoxazole, or pentomidine

Pulmonary embolism- Anticoagulant

Acute pulmonary edema- Patient develops acute breathlessness and cough productive of frothy and pink sputum. Patient cannot lie flat & on examination crackles are present both mid zones with scattered wheezes. Treat it with IV Frusemide.

Acute asthma attack- young patient presents with breathlessness and becomes too breathless to speak. There is tachycardia. Chest x ray may be normal. Treat with nebulized salbutamol.

Foreign body obstructing bronchial airway, patient is choked-Heimlich manoeuvre. Commonly observed that a person becomes suddenly breathless while eating and develops marked stridor, choking and drooling.

Pneumothorax and Pleural effusion- Needle aspiration. if recur, chest drain.

The common conditions should be kept in mind whenever any patient in ICU has chest problems, causes, investigations and treatment of choice:

1. Pneumonia- types of pneumonia, investigations, treatment of pnemonia

2. Hemoptysis- causes, investigations

3. Asthma- presentation, dignosis, treatment

4. Chest pain- causes, investigations, treatment

5. Breathlessness- causes, investigations

6. Pulmonary oedema- presentation, investigations, treatment

7. Cough- presentation, causes

8..Wheeze- investigation, treatment

9. Pleural effusion- presentation, investigations and treatment

Summary of Respiratory system

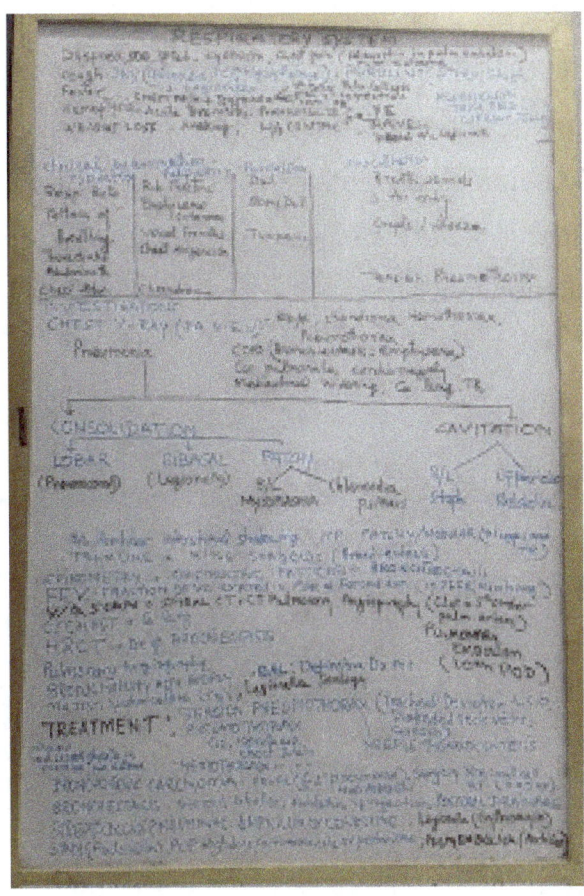

Mechanical Ventilation (Modes of Ventilators) in Intensive Care Unit (ICU)

Start your understanding about the setting of ventilators. The respiratory support to a patient by mechanical means, i.e., through machines (Ventilators) is known as Mechanical Ventilation). There are basically 3 modes of ventilation, i.e., CMV, SIMV and CPAP. Once youunderstand this, then it is very easy to know all about mechanical ventilation in ICU.

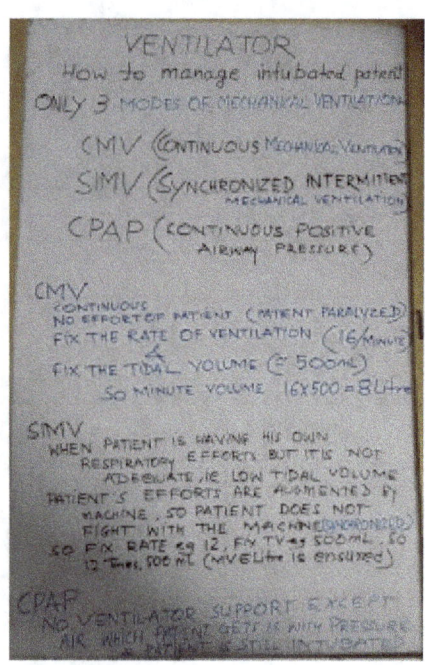

ABG (Arterial Blood Gas) Interpretation

Doctors, Nursing staff and Paramedical staff working in emergency & ICU setting need to know the value of ABG. It helps in the diagnosis of the conditions where a patient may require a correction of the electrolyte imbalance, respiratory problems and certain metabolic conditions and there may be requirement of mechanical ventilation.

Interpretation of ABG is very easy and one just need one page notes for interpretation of ABG. This image will make you confident of diagnosis of a patient who is on ventilator and may require some modification in the ventilator setting.

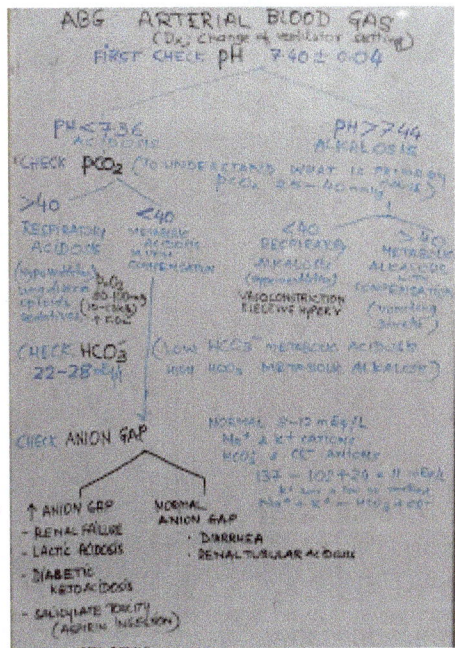

ANTIBIOTICS

Antibiotics are the medicines which are used to treat infections. Infections may be due to bacteria, fungus or virus. Almost everyone suffers from infection sometimes in life time especially in developing countries.

Being infected is a bad feeling and everybody dislikes it. Sometimes, these infections are so dreaded that it is better to get immunity against such bad infections. So, vaccines are used to present such bad infections, Commonly used vaccines are BCG (to prevent Tuberculosis), DPT (to prevent Diphtheria, Pertusis and Tetanus), Anti Hepatitis B Surface antigen Vaccine (to prevent infection against hepatitis B), Polio vaccine, etc.

But, all infections are not so dangerous, like common cold, sore throat, and small furuncle or small reddish pimple. Such infections usually subside by themselves due to the immunity of our own body. This immunity is mainly provided by white blood cells (WBCs) and lymphocytes present in our body. These act like Policemen patrolling our internal security. These security personnel detect and kill the foreign microbials or microorganisms like bacteria.

Sometimes, infecions may overwhelming and required to be treated with antibiotics. Like common cold not subsiding and persisting for longer duration with superadded bacterial infection or sinusitis. Or, sore throat associated with yellowish sputum with cough and fever. So, we need to take antibiotics to treat such infections.

Infections may be superficial or deep, local or systemic. The infection depends upon virulence or the microorganism, resistance of the person, and living conditions. Like persons with diabetes with uncontrolled blood sugar level and patients on long term steroids have low resistance or immunity against the infecive microrganisms. Person living in crowded places with other people infected with communicable diseases are prone to acquire infections of the airborne diseases like tuberculosis, influenza, etc.

Skin infections are commonly caused by Staphylococcus aureus and Streptococcus.

Invention of Penicillins in 1928 by Scottish researcher, Alexander Flemming, made a great difference to the outcome of patients with infections.

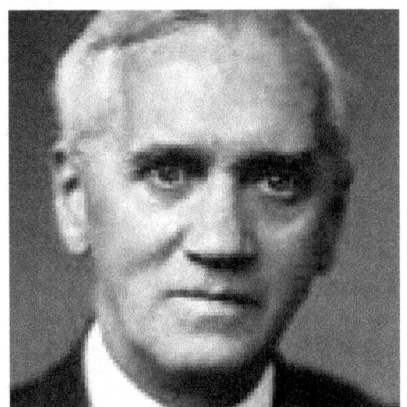

Sir Alexander Fleming

Sir Alexander Fleming was a Scottish physician, microbiologist, and pharmacologist. His best-known discoveries are the enzyme lysozyme in 1923 and the world's first antibiotic substance benzylpenicillin from the mould Penicillium notatum in 1928. The simple discovery and use of the antibiotic agent has saved millions of lives, and earned Fleming – together with Howard Florey and Ernst Chain, who devised methods for the large-scale isolation and production of penicillin – the 1945 Nobel Prize in Physiology/Medicine.

Penicillin was effective against fatal infections caused by bacteria. But, over time, these bacteria outsmarted the drug and developed resistance to these drugs. But, consistent efforts by the physicians, microbiologists, pharmacologists, biotechnologists and other inventors led to the development of many anti-microbial drugs which are commonly known as antibiotics.

So, commonly uses antibiotics are penicillins, cephalosporins, tetracyclines, macrolides, quinolones, anti-viral drugs, anti-fungal drugs, etc.

Common bacteria are described as Gram positive or Gram-negative. Gram positive bacteria are stained positively by Gram stain.

Some bacteria produce exotoxins and some produce endotoxins.

Tbe bacteria which produce exotoxins are Cornyebacterium diphtheriae, Clostridium tetani, C.botulinum, C.perfringens, Bacillus anthracis, Staphylococcus aureus, Streptococcus pogens (all are examples of Gram positive bacteria).

Gram negative bugs which produce exotoxins are E.coli, Vibrio cholerae, and Bordetella pertusis.

Endotoxin is a polysaccharide and is found in the cell wall of Gram-negative bacteria.

Some bacteria do not stain well with Gram-stain, like Treponema, Rickettsia, Mycoplasma, Legionella pneuophila, Mycobacteria and Chlamydia.

For treponemes-darkfield microscopy and fluorescent antibody staining is used.

Mycobacteria are acid-fast bacilli. Legionella is stained with silver stain.

Gram positive bacteria are broadly classified in 2 groups; Cocci and Bacilli.

Gram positive cocci are classified into two; catalase positive clusters (Staphylococcus) and catalase negative chains (Streptococcus).

Catalase postive staphylococci are further classified into two groups as Coagulase positive (S.aureus) and coagulase negative [Staphylococcus epidermidis (Novobiocin sensitive) and Staphylococcus saprophyticus (Novobiocin resistant].

Gram postive and catalase negative chains of cocci are Strptococcus. On the basis of hemolysis Streptococci are divided into 3 categories: Green (partial) hemolysis; Sterptococcus pneumoniae, Clear hemolysis Streptococcus pyogens (group A Bacitracin sensitive), S.agalactiae (group B, Bacitracin resistant) and 3rd category of streptococci with no hemolysis examples are Enterococcus (E.fecalis) and Peptostreptococcus(anaerobe).

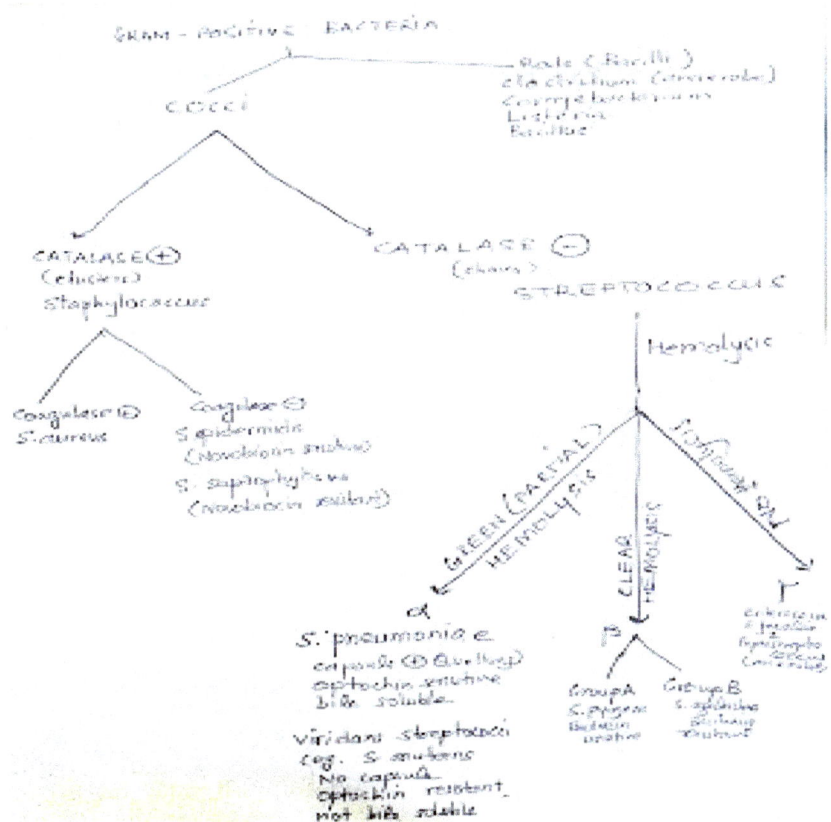

Exapmple of Gram positive bacilli (rods) are: Clostridium (anaerobe), Cornyebacterium, Listeria and Bacillus.

Gram negative bacteria which appear pink are broadly classified into three groups : Cocci, C0ccoid rods and rods.

Gram negative cocci are Neisseria mningitidis and N.gonorrhoeae. These two are differentiated on the basis of Maltose fermenter chacteristic. N. menigitidis is Malose fermenter and N. gonorrhoeae is Maltose noferenter.

The examples of cgram negative coccoid rods are Hemophlus influenzae, Pasteurella, Brucella and Bordetella pertusis.

Gram negative rods are further subdivided into two subtypes based Lactose fermenter characteristic. Lactose fermenter gram negative rods are Klebsiella, E,coli and Enterobacter which are Fast fermenter and Citrobacter, and Serratia Slow fermenters.

Lactose nonfermenter gram negative rods are subdivided into two groups, based on oxidase property. Oxidase positive are Pseudomonas and oxidase negative are Shigella, Salmonella and Proteus.

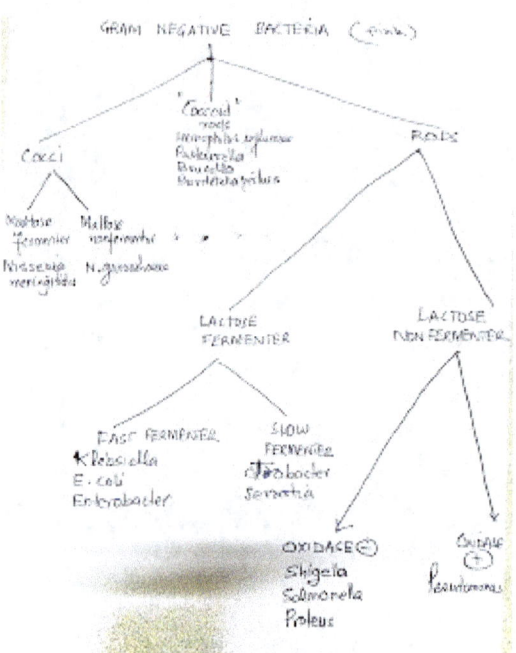

Penicillin C is for intravenous use and Penicillin V is for oral use.

Penicillin binds penicillin-binding proreins , blocks transpeptidase cross-linking of cell wall and activates autolytic enzymes. It is bactericidal for gram positive cocci and rods, gram negative cocci and spirochetes.

Methicillin, nafcillin have narrow spectrum and used against penicillase resistant Staphyloccus aureus.

Ampicillin, Amoxicillin have wider spectrum, penicillanse sensitive, also combined with clavulanic acid (penicillanase inhibitor) to enhance spectrum. Amoxicillin has greater oral bioavailability than ampicillin. These two extended-spectrum penicillin and are useful against certain gram positive bacteria and gram negative rods (Hemophilus influenzae, E.coli, Listeria monocytogens, Proteus mirabilis, Salmonella and enterococci).

Carbenicillin, Piperacillin and Ticarcillin are extended spectrum penicillin and useful against Pseudomonas and gram negative rods , susceptible to penicillanase, used with clavulanic acid.

Cephalosporins are beta lactam drugs. It inhibits cell wall synthesis

Imipenem

Imipenem is a broad spectrum, beta lactamase-resistant carbapenem. It is always administered with cilastatin which is inhibitor of renal dihydropeptidase 1 to decrease inactivation in renal tubules. Ii is used against gram positive cocci, gram negative rods and anaerobes. It is drug of hoice against Enterobacter. Its toxicity includes GI distress, skin rash, and CNS oxicity (seizures).

The important group of antibiotics which are commonly used in neurosurgical practice are:

Vancomycin

Aminoglycosides

Tetracyclines

Macrolides

Chloramphenicol

Clindamycin

Sulfonamides

Trimethoprim

Fluroquinolones

Metronidazole

References:

Wikpedia

Alexander Fleming (1881–1955): Discoverer of penicillin, Siang Yong Tan, Yvonne Tatsumura

Singapore Med J. 2015 Jul; 56(7): 366–367. doi: 10.11622/smedj.2015105

Thorough Neurological Examination- All in One Page

Never ever presume a neurological diagnosis without interacting with a patient and just by seeing the radiology report or just by listening the patient's complaints. Examine a patient without any presumption & bias, You will always feel rewarded. Listen to the patient. Patient is the best guide and will provide you the important clue for the diagnosis. History taking is an opportunity to interact with people from diversified background.

While taking history of a patient who is suspected to have a neurological disorder it should always be prudent to take history pertaining to lesions of brain, spinal cord and peripheral nerves. In this manner you can complete and cover the entire central and peripheral nervous system.

So, if you suspect a lesion of the cerebral hemisheres, History of Seizure, Headache, Vision and , Deterioration of conscious level or loss of consciousness, Weakness of the face or limbs should be taken into detail.

If you suspect a lesion of cerebellum, then history of imbalance, ataxia and difficulty in walking should always be taken.

And if you suspect a lesion of the brain stem (Midbrain , pons, medulla Oblongata), the symptoms of multiple cranial nerve deficits (speech abnormality, nystagmus, difficulty in deglutition, loss of Gag reflex), and long tract signs (weakness in limbs, hyperrelexia, increased tone in limbs, positive Babinski sign) are expected.

In patients with lesions of the spinal cord history must include details about weakness of the limbs, bladder and bowel involvement.

History of ==headache== must include Onset (sudden, gradual), Site (holocranial, hemicranial , temoral)Frequency, duration, severity, Character (Aching, throbbing), timing (e.g., morning , evening), Precipitating factors (coughing, strenuous work) , Relieving factors (analgesics, rest) , Associated features (nausea, vomiting, visual disturbance).

History of ==Visual Disorder== should include onset, frequency, impairment (uniocular or both eyes, partial or total), diplopia, Precipitaing factor, Associated features

History of ==Loss of Consciousness== may be due to syncope because of cardiac causes or vasovagal shock or due to neurological causes like a part of seizure or neurotrauma or a space occupying lesion in the brain. Loss of consciousness may also be due to low blood sugar level in a patient on diabetic treatment or alcohol or drug abuse.

Speech disorder may be a difficulty in Articulation or Expression or Understanding.

Weakness in the limbs may be Quadriparesis, Hemiparesis or Monoparesis with or without involvement of facial muscles.

History of **Sensory system abnormalities** may expressed by the patient as Numbness, feeling of crawling of ants or insects, Tingling or inability to feel a part of the body.

History of **cranial nerve deficits** may be expressed by the patient as inability to smell, inability to read, loss of vision, diplopia, frequent changes of spectacle, partial closure of the eyelid (Ptosis)loss of sensation over the face, drooling of saliva from the side, difficulty in closing eye, slurring of speech or change in voice, difficulty in hearing or Deafness, Tinnitus, Vertigo or Dizziness, inability to swallow, inability to shrug and turn face and inability to protrude tongue.

Neurological examination is straight forward, It is like substraction and addition of numbers, like 2+2=4. So, if there is right hemiparesis of body and face and the deep tendon reflexes are increaded, there must be some lesion on the left side of the brain. There is nothing wrong in rechecking the neurological examination findings. But, be sure of your neurological examination findings. Your examination may have a great impact on clinical outcome and plan of the treatment. In Neuroscience most of the things are evident. As students we used to think that many things may be theortical. But, with the advent of newer and advanced neuroradiology, microneurosurgery and functional neurosurgery, lot of procedures are now based on physiological and neuroanatomical localization.

One should begin with systemic examination. See Pallor (anemia), Icterus (jaundice), Lymhadenopathy. Anemia may explain many symptoms.

Lymhadenopathy may indicate infection, lymphoma or metastasis.

Examine Pulse: Bradycardia is an omnious sign of raised intrcranial pressure (ICP)
                Irregular Pulse may indicate syncope

Blood pressure : Hypertension may indiacte raise ICP

Respiratory Rate: Irregular Respiration, Bradycardia and Hypertension are parts of Cushing reflex which is due to raised ICP.

Neck rigidity may indicate meningitis or subarachnoid hemorrhage. Restriction of neck movement may be due to cervical spondylosis. One should be very careful while examining a patient with head injury. if a patient is unconscious and his GCS is 8 or less, it is presumed that there may be associated cervical spine injury. So, in severely head injured patient, neck should be immobilized by putting a cervical collar while shifting the patient

Neurological examination begins with higher mental function. orientation to time, place and person should be asked.

cranial nerve examination: Soap may be used to examine olfaction. Vision should be seen in both eyes. If patient is unable to count fingers, then perception of light should be examined with a torch. Pupillary light reflex,ie, constrction of both the pupils when light is projected in eye, gives a clue about both second and third cranial nerves. because second cranial nerve (Optic Nerve) is afferent and third cranial nerve (Occulomotor nerve) is efferent of this light reflex. Although this is very simple examination but it has great value. We often presume that vision is normal and miss it. A child with craniopharyngima, an adult with clinodal meningima or pituitary adenoma may not have any vision in one eye but even patiets or their parents may not be aware about the uniocular visual loss. So, if a doctor misses this finding, there may be catastrophic consequences. As immediately following the surgery, there is natural tendency in everyone to check the vision and it could be concluded that this visual loss be due to surgery. Optic nerve tumor, optic nerve injury, retinal detachmentmay also present with uniocular visual loss.

3,4,6 cranial nerves function may be examined by seeing the conjugate eye movements of both eyes together.

5th cranial nerve, 7th cranial nerve is by examining the face. sensation over the face is mainly by the Vth cranial nerve (Trigeminal nerve). There are three sensory divisions of Trigeminal nerve (V1, V2, V3). 7th cranial nerve is the motor supply to the face.

Hearing is through 8th cranial nerve. Ideally 8th cranial nerves should be examined by Tuning forks. If patient hears the rubbing of fingers of the examiner close to each ear, it may give some clue to the intact hearing.

If the gag reflex is intact, 9th and 10th cranial nerves are intact.

Patient is asked to Shrug the shoulder and turn the face against the resistance to examine sternocleidomastoid and trapezius muscle which are suppled by the spinal accessory nerve.

Protrusion of tongue is possible with the 12th cranial nerve. If Hypoglossal nerve is damaged the tongue deviates to the injured side on protruding.

Sensory nervous examination should be done before motor examination. Because patients usually are cooperative and sensory system examination is subjective and needs patient,s cooperation.

Motor examination : Movement of all four limbs. Power in all four limbs should be checked separately and should be compared with your own strength. Deep tendon reflexes and tone should also be examined.

Gait; If a patient is able to walk, gait should also be examined to complete the thorough neurological examination

Neurosurgery is a new subspeciality of surgery with a very little progress in terms of clinical outcome despite of lot of technological advancements in last few decades. Neurosurgical management has greatly been helped by advancements in neuroradiology like CT scan, MRI, and angiography. Very little progress has been witnessed over the innovative surgical skills and clinical outcome as reported during the period of Victor Horsley, Harvey Cushing and Walter Dandy about a century ago. As a trainee there is a need to have a bird eye view of the whole gamut of neurosurgery including Gamma knife, functional neurosurgery, neuro intervention, apart from learning skills of skull base neurosurgery, vascular neurosurgery, spinal instrumentation, repair of nerve injuries, surgery for craniosynostosis, spinal dysraphism, encephaloceles and neuroendoscopy. Some neurosurgical centers may not have expertise and facilities for providing comprehensive teaching and training in neurosurgery.

Neurosurgery resident doctors should have the basic concepts of the neurosurgical procedures. The neurosurgery can broadly be classified as cranial neurosurgery, spinal neurosurgery and peripheral neurosurgery. There are different subspecialitiies of neurosurgery like pediatric neurosurgery, functional neurosurgery, neuro-oncology, spinal neurosurgery, skull base neurosurgery, vascular neurosurgery, endoscopic neurosurgery, stereotactic neurosurgery, neurointervention, etc.

So, there is a whole range of procedures in neurosurgery and it requires a resident doctors to have atleast some idea about these procedures.

Basic Neuroanatomy for the Beginner (Brain, Spinal cord and Nerves)
Broadly speaking, brain is the anatomical structure and mind is the physiological (functional) component.
In another simple manner, brain can be described as the hardware like a computer hardware and mind can be described as the software of a computer.

When we talk about Neuroanatomy then it means study of the brain, spinal cord, cranial nerves, spinal nerves, nerve plexuses, dermatomes, muscles and joints supplied by these nerves. At the outset it seems very tough to master neuroanatomy, but it is very interesting and easy to learn.

Functionally, the nervous system is divided into the somatic nervous system, which controls the voluntary activites and the visceral (autonomic) nervous system, which controls involuntary activities.

Anatomically, the nervous system can be divided into 2 subdivisions:
CNS (Central Nervous System) & PNS (Peripheral Nervous System).

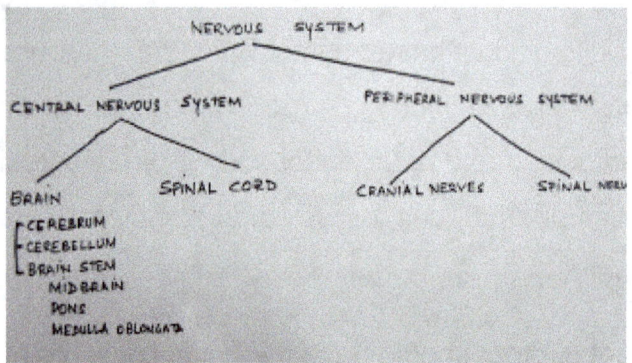

CNS consists of brain & spinal cord.
PNS consists of cranial nerves & spinal nerves. The peripheral nervous system consists of 12 pairs of cranial nerves and 31 pairs of spinal nerves, and their associated ganglia.

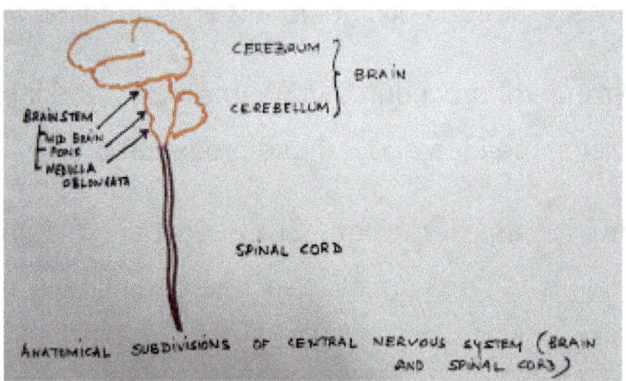

As the basic building materials of a house are brick and cement, similarly the Nervous system is made by the Neurons and Neuroglia.
Neuron is the basic unit of nervous system.
Neuroglia are non-neuronal cells and these are of three types: Astrocytes, Oligodendrocytes and Microglia.

Neuron or nerve cell is the basic functional unit of the nervous system. There are about 100 billion neurons in central nerovous system. They are supported by glial cells. They are present in brain and spinal cord and glial cells outnumber neurons (10:1).

Neurons are the structural and functional units of the nervous system.
Neuronons consist of cell bodies (perikaryon or soma) with dendrites and axon.
Dendrites (dendron means tree) are short and highly branched and carry impulses toward the cell body.
Axons are usually single and long, have fewer branches (collaterals), and carry impulses away from the cell body.
Myelin is the fat like substance forming a sheath around the axons of certain nerve fibers. It is formed by Schwann cells in the PNS and oligodendrocytes in the CNS.

Neuroglial cells or Glial cells are of three types: astrocytes, oligodendrocytes and microglia. Astrocytes and Oligodendrocytes can be classified together as Macroglia. Macroglia is dervived from ectoderm. Astrocytes regulate the ionic environment & reuptake of neurotransmitters. They form the blood brain barrier. There are two broad classes of astrocytes: protoplasmic and fibrous. Astrocytes provide structural support to nervous tissue and act during development as guidewires that direct neuronal migration. They also maintain appropriate concentration of ions such as Potassium ions within the extracelluar space of brain & spinal cord.
Astrocytes form a covering on the entire CNS surface & proliferate to aid in repairing to aid in repairing damaged neural tissue. These reactive astrocytes are larger, are more easily stained, and can be identified in histological sections because they contain a characteristic, astrocyte-specific protein: glial fibrillary acidic protein (GFAP). Chronic astrocytic proliferation leads to gliosis, sometimes called glial scarring.
Oligodendrocytes form the myelin sheath around neurons in central nervous system. (In peripheral nervous system , i.e., in case of spinal nerves, the Myelin sheath is formed by the Schwannn cells).
Oligodendrocytes predominate in white matter; they extend arm-like processes which wrap tightly around axons.
Microglia or microglial cells are the macrophages or scavengers of the CNS & do the

immune surveillance of the CNS.

Nerve cells convey signals to one another at synapses. Chemical transmitters (or Neurotransmitters) are associated with the function of the synapse: excitation or inhibition. A neuron may receive thousands of synapses, which bring in information from many sources.

Brain anatomy can be described under following headings: cerebrum, cerebellum and brainstem. Cerebrum consists of two cerebral hemispheres which are connected to each other with commissural fibers. The largest bundle of commissural fibers is corpus callosum, which connects the two cerebral hemispheres.

Cerebellum is situated on posterior aspect of brain, below the cerebrum and behind brain stem

Brain stem comprises Midbrain, Pons and Medulla oblongata.

Brain constitutes about 2% of the body weight but receives about 18-20% of cardiac output. It controls all the functions of the body. It is of great interest to everyone. The human brain is very much different from the brain of other creatures in view of its immense capacity. A large surface area of the neural tissue is contained inside the cranium or skull. It is possible because of large number of infoldings which take the shape of sulci and gyri. The part which caves in is called the sulcus and the elevated part is called gyrus.
The neuroanatomy is very interesting and lot of advancements have occurred in the understanding of the microneurosurgical anatomy of the brain.
Almost all body parts of the body are represented in the cerebral hemispheres. Different areas of the cerebral hemisheres have been assigned different functions.

Three membranes cover the brain and spinal cord, these are known as meninges. The innermost is Piamater, middle layer is Arachnoid layer and the outermost is the thickest layer, the Duramater. The Dura is also called the pachymeninx, and the arachnoid and pia are called the leptomeninges. the dura mater is tough, fibrous sheath and is continuous with the spinal dura.

The arachnoid is a thin, transparent sheath separated from the underlying pia by the subarachnoid space, which contains cerebrospinal fluid (CSF).

Brain floats inside a fluid called cerebrospinal fluid (CSF). CSF is contained between Arachnoid layer and Piamater.

Cerebral hemispheres, corpus callosum, brain stem , cerebellum are contained inside a hard bony structure known as cranium or skull. To protect the soft brain against the hard bony structures, there are wide CSF spaces at the base of the brain, known as CSF Cisterns.

Spinal cord is contained in the vertebral column or spine. Spinal cord is about 45 centimeter in length and about 30 grams in weight. Spinal cord is continuous with the medulla at its upper end. Conus medullaris is the lower or inferior end of the spinal cord.In adults, the conus ends at the lower border of the L1 vertebra.
Brain and spinal cord together is known as central nervous system. The cranial nerves and spinal nerves constitute the peripheral nervous system.

Brain is situated inside the skull or cranium.

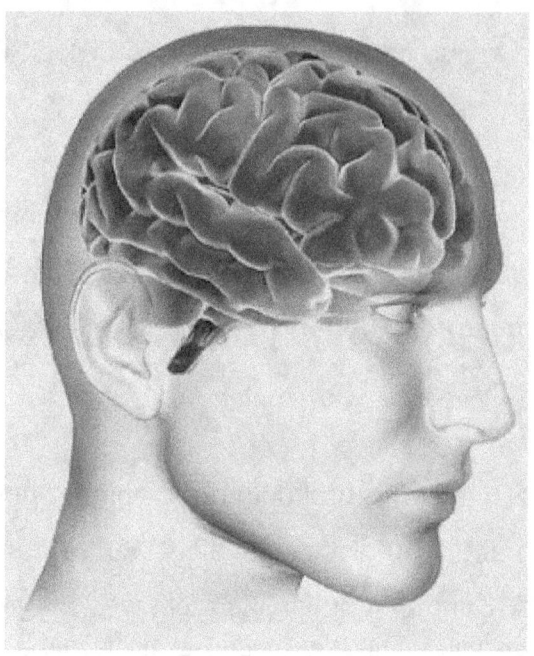

Weight of brain in an adult is about 1,300 - 1,400 Grams (Approximately 1.4 kg).

Weight of brain in a newborn is about 350 - 400 Grams.

Brain constitutes 2% of total body weight.

Intracranial contents by volume (1,700 ml, 100%):
- brain = 1,400 ml (80%);
- blood = 150 ml (10%);
- cerebrospinal fluid = 150 ml (10%)

Average number of neurons in the brain = 100 billion

Average number of glial cells in brain = 10-50 times the number of neurons

Rate of production of CSF = 0.35 ml/min (500 ml/day)

% blood flow from heart to brain = 15-20%

Blood flow through whole brain (adult) = 750 ml/min

% brain utilization of total resting oxygen = 20%

Cerebral blood flow = 55 ml/100 g brain tissue/min

Cerebral cortex on surface can be divided into four major lobes- Frontal, Parietal, Temporal and Occipital Lobes.

To summarise, the weight of brain in an adult is approximately 1.4 kg and it appears as a soft structure. It is covered inside three coverings : the outermost layer is called duramater, the middle layer is called Arachnoid layer and the innermost layer is Pia mater. In between Arachnoid and Pia mater there is a space called Subarachnoid space which contains Cerebrospinal fluid (CSF).

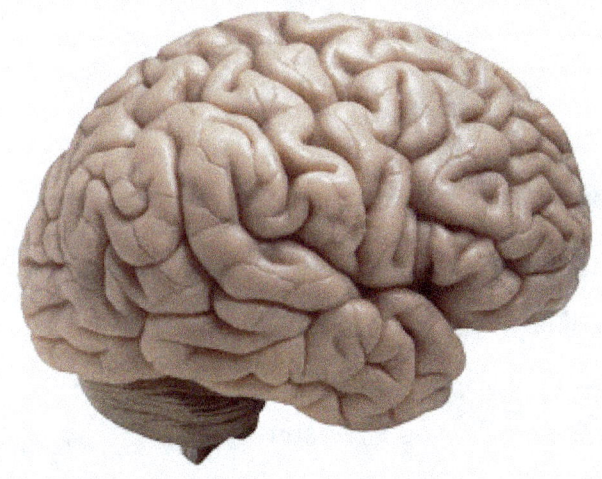

(Fig Source: www.shortfacts.com)

The cadaveric brain without blood vessels looks like this picture. It has various infoldings which increase the surface area of the brain. There are various sulci and gyri.

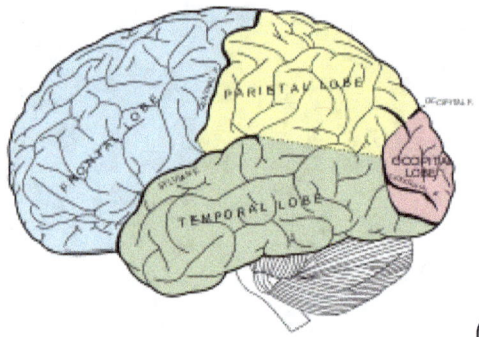

(Fig source en.wikipedia.org)

The brain components can be understood in a very simple way as this picture. The large part above is called Cerebraum and posterior and lower part is called Cerebellum.

Cerebrum consists of two cerebral hemispheres.

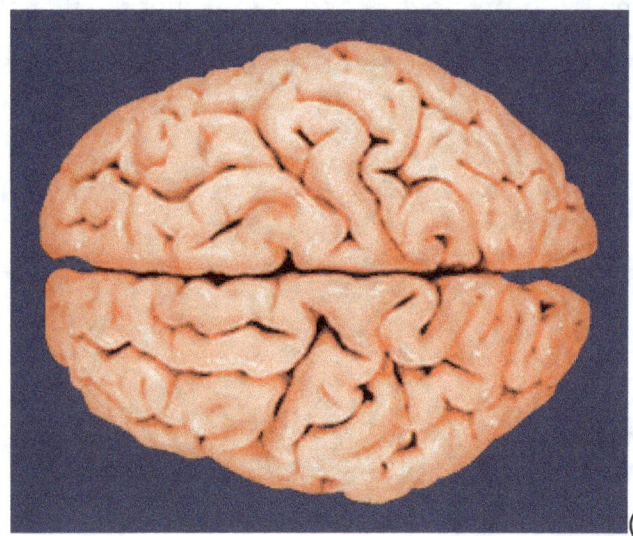

(Fig Source Morphonix)

Each cerebral hemisphere can be divided into Frontal, Parietal , temporal and Occipital Lobe.

The two cerebral hemispheres are connected in the midline with a bundle of commissural fibers known as Corpus Callosum.

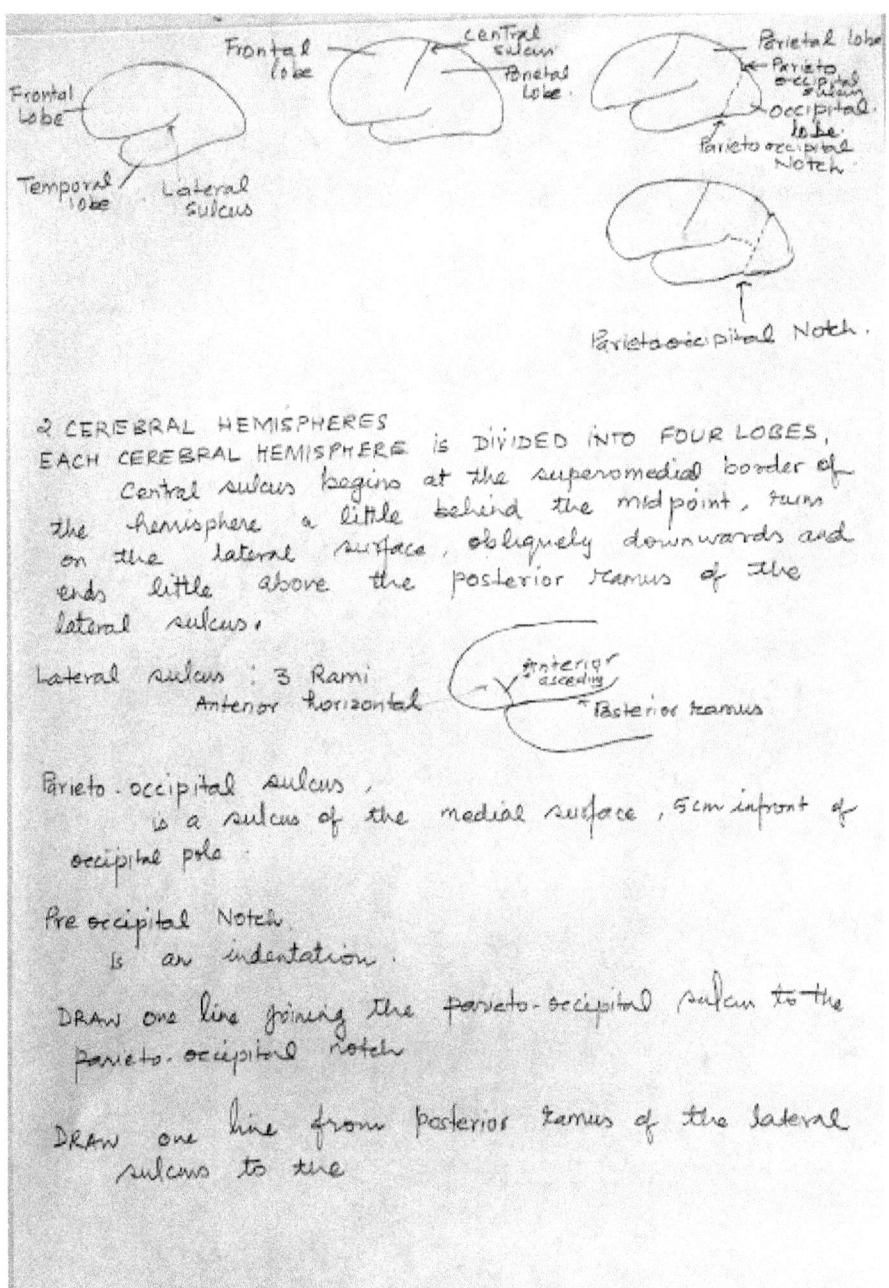

To understand neuroanatomy, one should begin with practice of drawing lateral surface of the brain.

So, the easiest way is to draw this diagram. An elliptical shape with a line. This diagram helps to know the boundary between frontal lobe and temporal lobe of brain.

To understand neuroanatomy, one should begin with practice of drawing lateral surface of the brain.

So, the easiest way is to draw this diagram. An elliptical shape with a line. This diagram helps to know the boundary between frontal lobe and temporal lobe of brain.

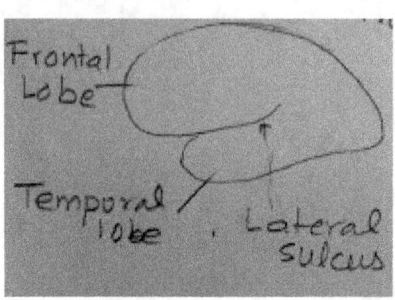

Then draw a line to show the central sulcus which separates frontal lobe and parietal lobe.

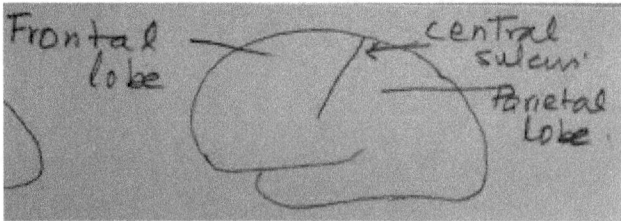

Then an imaginary line is drawn which connects the parieto-occipital sulcus to pre-occipital notch. Then another imaginary line is drawn from the posterior end of the sylvian fissure to the center of previous imaginary line connecting parieto-occipital sulcus to pre-occipital notch. .

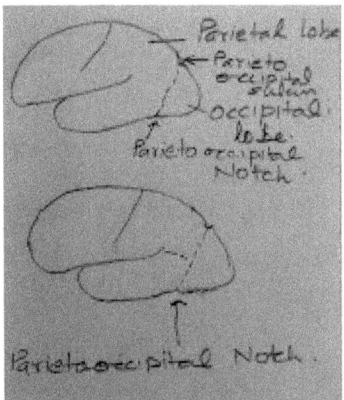

Now, the all 4 lobes of each cerebral hemispheres may be labelled, and their boundaries may be remembered.

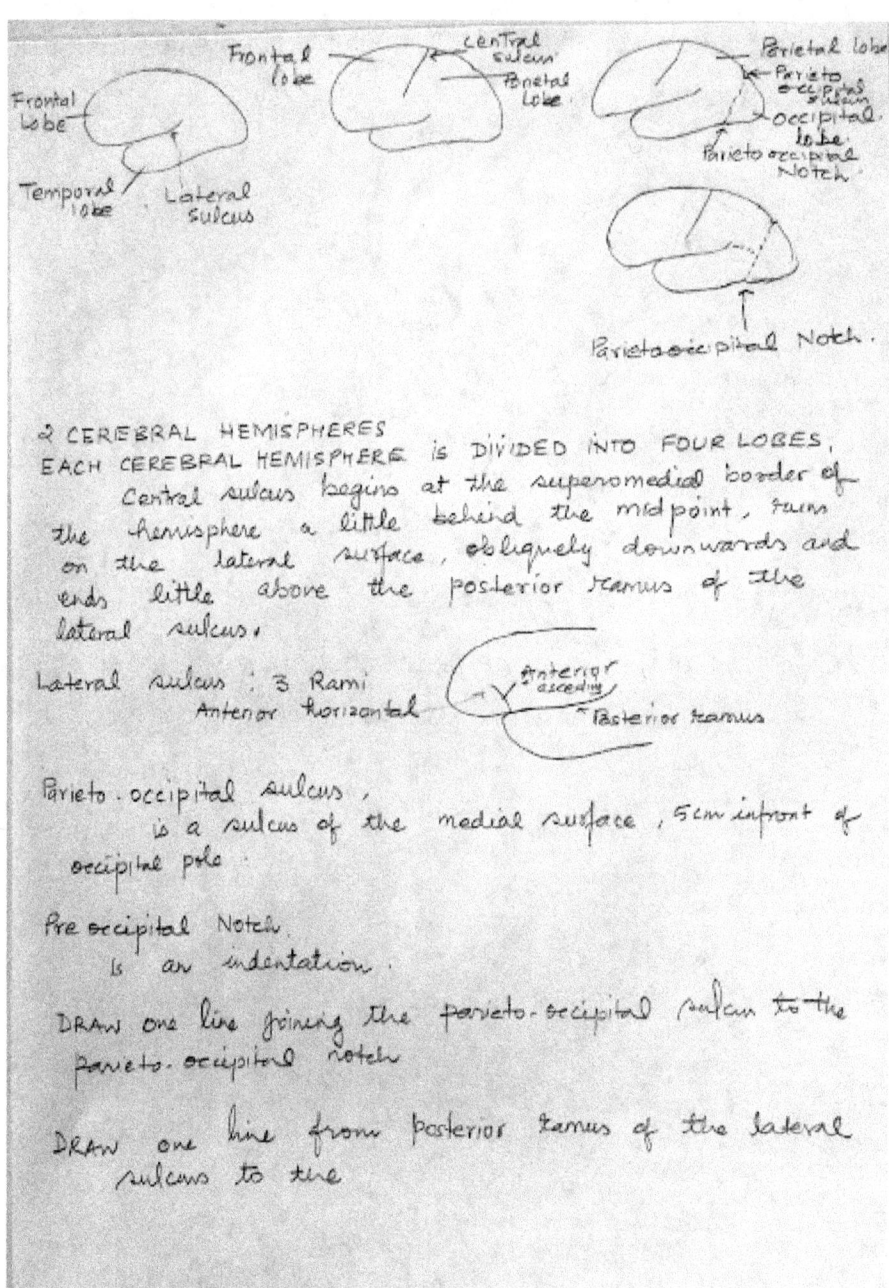

2 CEREBRAL HEMISPHERES
EACH CEREBRAL HEMISPHERE IS DIVIDED INTO FOUR LOBES.
Central sulcus begins at the superomedial border of the hemisphere a little behind the midpoint, turns on the lateral surface, obliquely downwards and ends little above the posterior ramus of the lateral sulcus.

Lateral sulcus: 3 Rami
  Anterior horizontal
  Anterior ascending
  Posterior ramus

Parieto-occipital sulcus.
  is a sulcus of the medial surface, 5cm infront of occipital pole.

Pre occipital Notch.
  is an indentation.

DRAW one line joining the parieto-occipital sulcus to the parieto-occipital notch

DRAW one line from posterior ramus of the lateral sulcus to the

Now, it is easy to understand about all the sulci and gyri over the lateral surface of cerebral hemispheres.

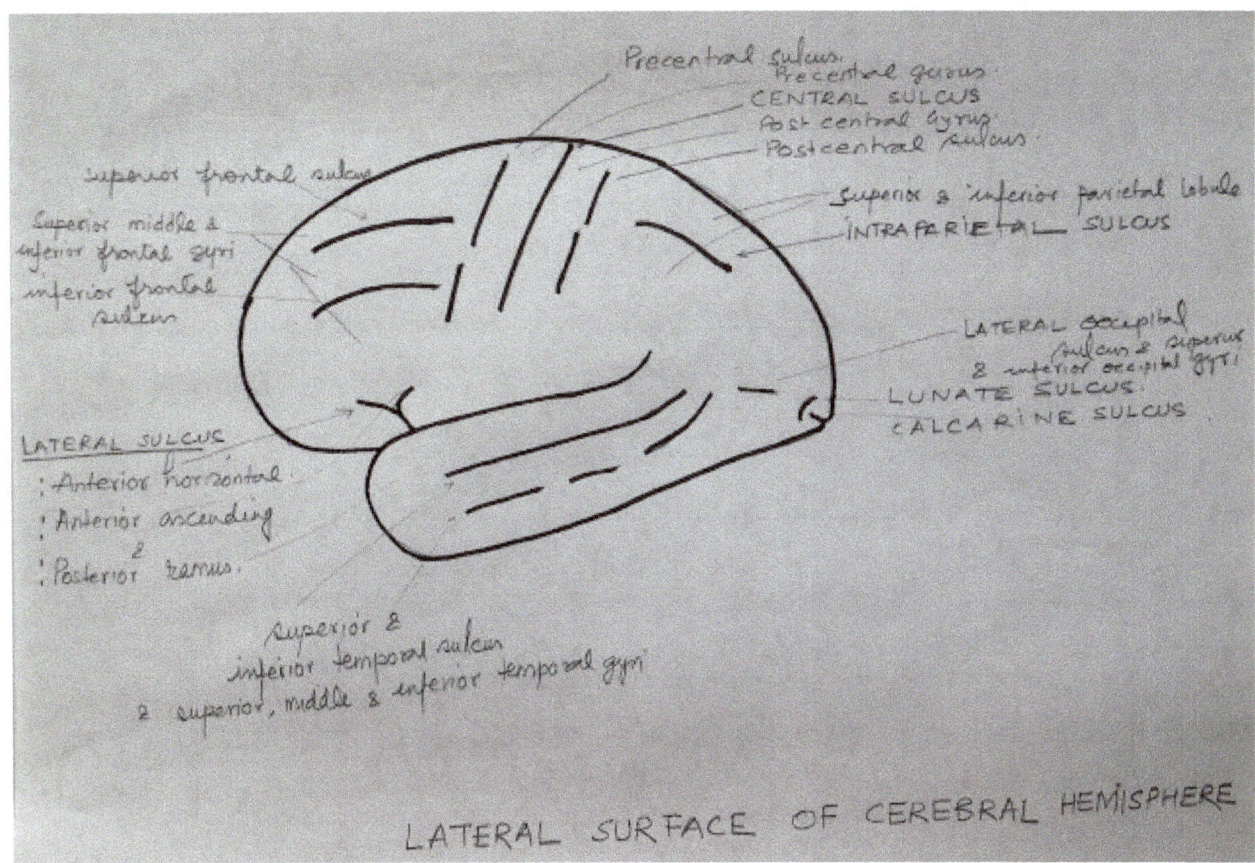

LATERAL SURFACE OF CEREBRAL HEMISPHERE

BRODMANN'S AREAS

As you know that almost all areas of the body are represented in the cerebral hemisphere which are known as Brodmann,s areas. These areas are given different numbers. Like Motor area, Sensory area, Speech area, visual area, hearing area. Important functional areas of brain are :

Primary Motor area or Primary Motor Cortex or Motor Strip or Precentral Gyrus (area 4)

Primary Somatosensory cortex (areas 3,1,2 are situated in the post central gyrus, i.e. part of the Parietal lobe just posterior to the central sulcus)

Primary auditory area or Transverse gyrus of Heschl (areas 41 & 42)

Broca's Speech Area (area 44) is situated in the dominant inferior frontal gyrus which is usually left inferior frontal gyrus in right handed person.

Wernicke's area (Receptive speech area)

Frontal eye field (area 8)

Primary Visual Cortex (area 17)

Various images of the brain is available on the internet, I have chosen a few for you so that you may have an idea about the orientation of parts of brain and spinal cord

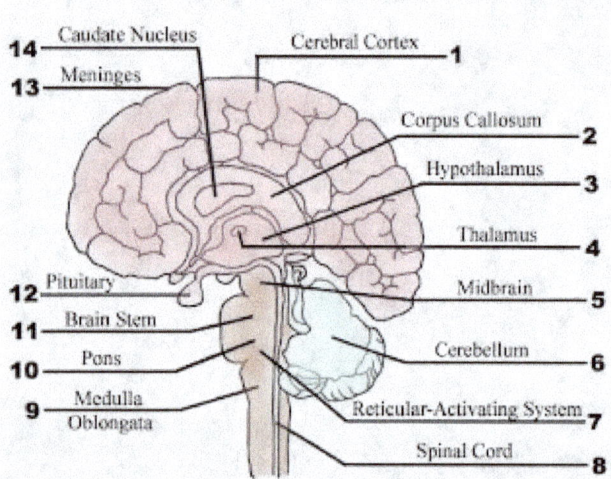

This figure simplifies the various parts inside the brain . The cerebrum and cerebellum are situated on the stem , known as brain stem. Brain Stem consists of Mid Brain, Pons and Medulla Oblongata.

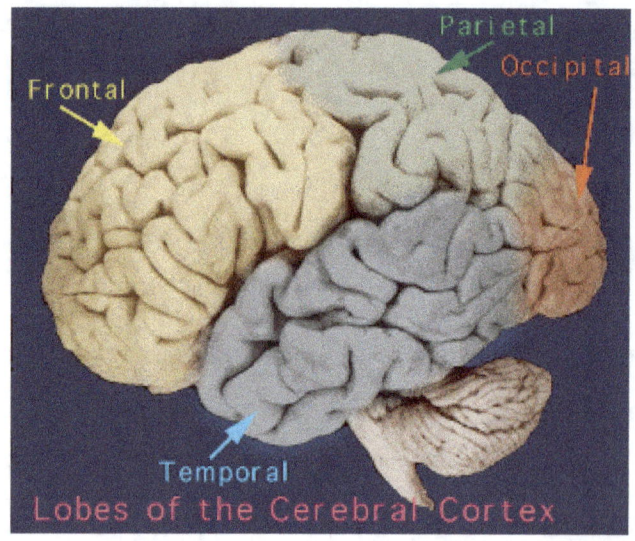

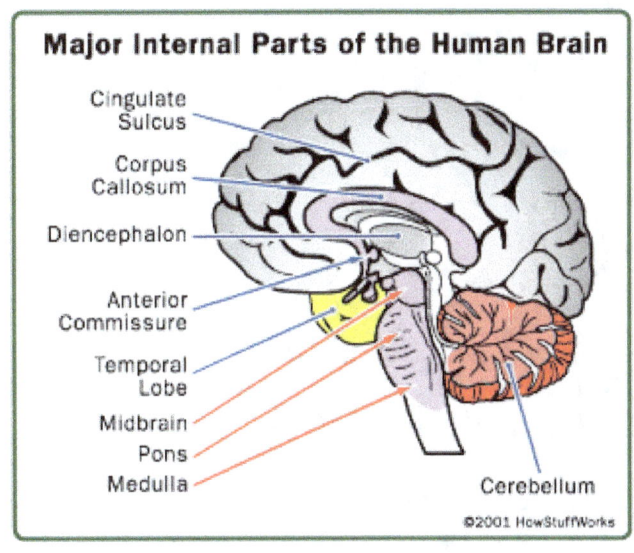

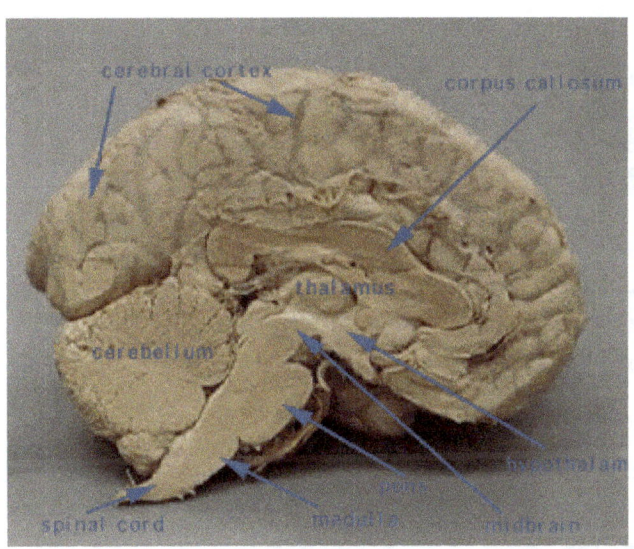

Actual look of a sagittal section of brain of a human cadaver showing Mid sagittal structures of the brain. An understading of this picture will help you to read a sagittal image of the MI of the brain. It shows corpus callosum, cerebellum, Midbrain, Pons and Medulla Oblongata. Corpus callosum connects two cerebral hemisheres.

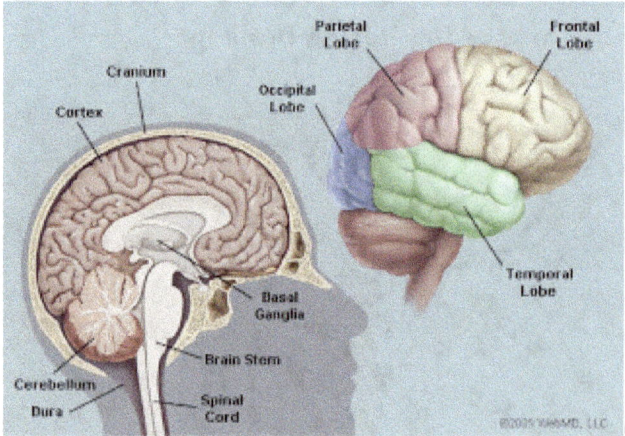
(Fig source: www.webmd.com)

This picture gives an idea about the skull (Cranium), brain (Cerbral hemispheres and Cerebellum), and spinal cord.

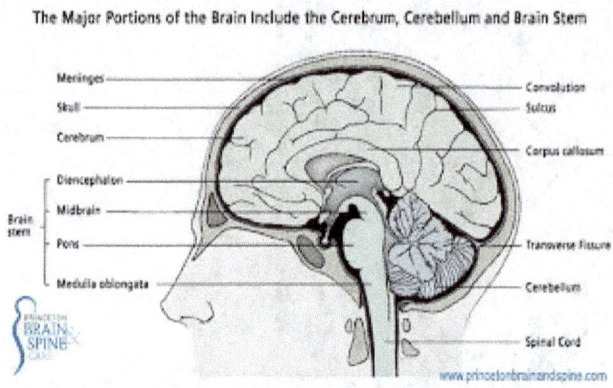

It is the mid sagittal section image : Below the corpus callosum is lateral ventricle and below the Fornix is third ventricle . The Floor of the third ventricle shows pituitary stalk. This picture gives an idea about the relation of the brain to the orbit, location of pituitary gland to the nasal cavity, location of the brain stem.

If someone has an idea about the axial , coronal and sagittal sections of the brain it becomes easy to interpret the CT scan and MRI of the brain.

Spinal cord is the continuation of the lower part of brain stem, i.e., medulla oblongata. Medulla oblongata ends at foramen magnum, i.e., an opening at the posterior end of skull.

Almost all the functions are regulated by the brain and some examples are motor function, speech, vision,etc. Different areas of the brain regulate different functions.

Arterial supply of the brain can be described as anterior circulation and posterior circulation. the anterior circulation is contributed by internal carotid artery and posterior circulation is contributed by vertebral arteries. Internal carotid artery is branch of common carotid artery and vertebral artery is a branch of subclavian artery.

The vertebral arterial system supplies the brain stem, cerebellum, parts of thalamus. The internal carotid artery supplies blood to remainder of the brain (about 85%). Circle of Willis is a circle of arteries at the base of the brain that gives rise to all the major blood supply to the brain. The circle of Willis is named after the English neuroanatomist Sir Thomas Willis. It is formed by two anterior cerebral arteries which are in communication with each other anteriorly through one anterior communicating artery. There are two posterior communicating arteries which are connected to the posterior cerebral arteries, the terminal branches of basilar artery.

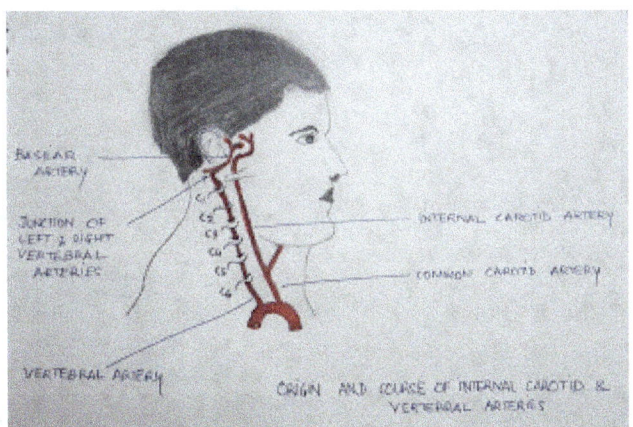

This image simplifies the concept of blood supply of the brain. Two Internal carotid arteries (ICA) and two vertebral arteries supply the arterial blood to whole brain. About 85% of blood supply comes from ICA and it constitutes anterior circulation, remaining 15% comes from vertebral artery which contributes to posterior circulation. This image also shows the course of vertebral artery which travrses through the foramen transversorium (an opening in the transverse process of C1 to C6 cervical vertebrae, the transverse process of C7 vertebra has only rudimentary opening) of C1 to C6 cervical vertebrae and enters the cranium through the Foramen Magnum, from posterior to anterior, and two vertebral arteries join to form Basilar Artery in front of the Pons. Basilar artery runs in midline, anterior to the Pons.

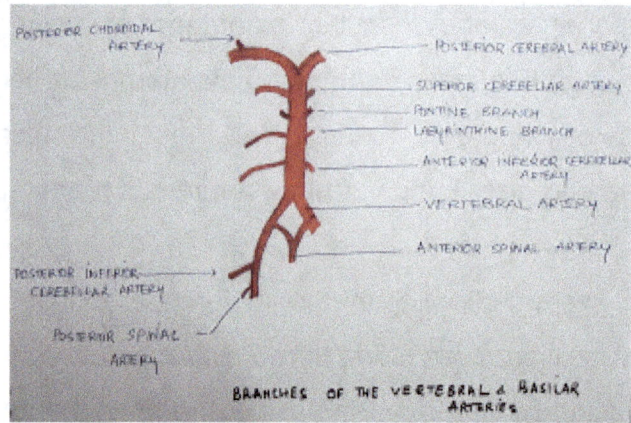

So, another image will be able to explain the entire blood supply of brain: How arteries arise from Arch of Aorta, Subclavian artery and formation of circle of Willis.

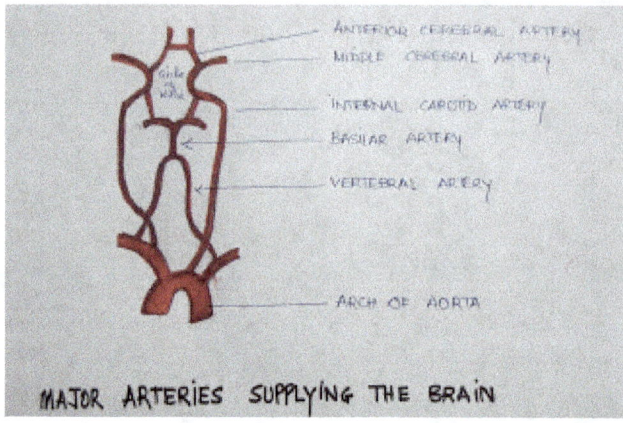

Venous system of brain

All the veins of the brain drain into Internal Jugular Vein which drains into right atrium of the heart. But the venous drainage of brain is different from other structures of the body. The veins of the brain can be described as superficial and deep venous systems of the brain.

Superficial venous system of the brain

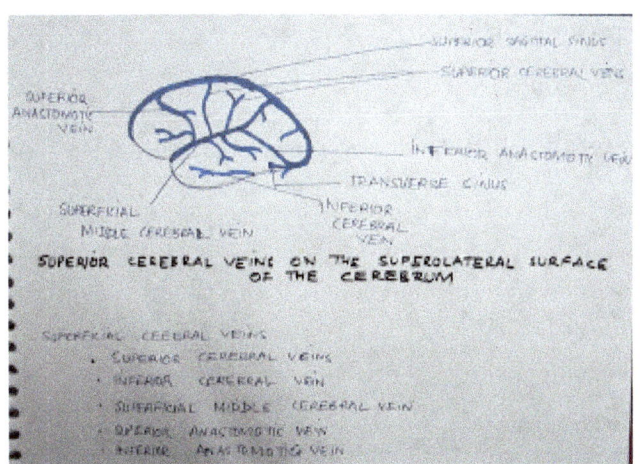

Deep Venous System of the Brain

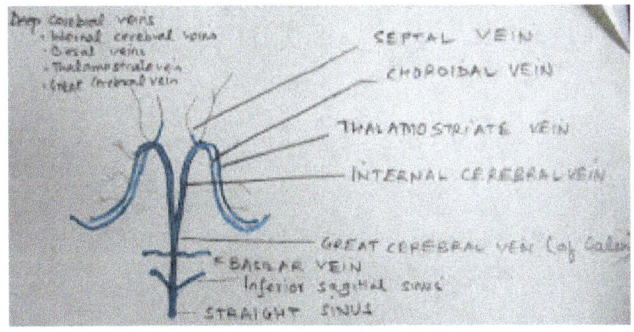

Cranial nerves

There are 12 pairs of cranial nerves

Cranial nerve I Olfactory nerve

Cranial nerve II Optic nerve

Cranial nerve III Oculomotor nerve

CN IV Trochlear nerve

CN V Trigeminal nerve

CN VI Abducens nerve

CN VII Facial nerve

CNVIII Vestibulocochlear nerve

CNI X Glossopharyngeal nrve

CN X Vagus nerve

CN XI Spinal Acessory nerve

CN XII Hypoglossal nerve

Cranial nerves 128 are sensory nerves, 5, 7, 9 and 10 are mixed nerves and rest are motor cranial nerves.

(So, to know the type of cranial nerves, remember just two numbers 128, and 5790).

Contrary to the popular belief about difficulty in neuroscience and brain anatomy, it is very easy to understand the neuroanatomy. If someone aims to master the neuroanatomy, the way is very simple. Begin with understanding the basic anatomy of skull, brain, vertebral column and spinal cord in a step wise manner. I have drawn the pictures of the skull, brain and spinal cord to highlight the value of these basic facts.

This manner of learning is good for the medical students and neurosurgeons as well. The ability to draw the image of a skull helps in understanding the parts of skull. This helps in understanding neuroradiology and in the surgical planning also.

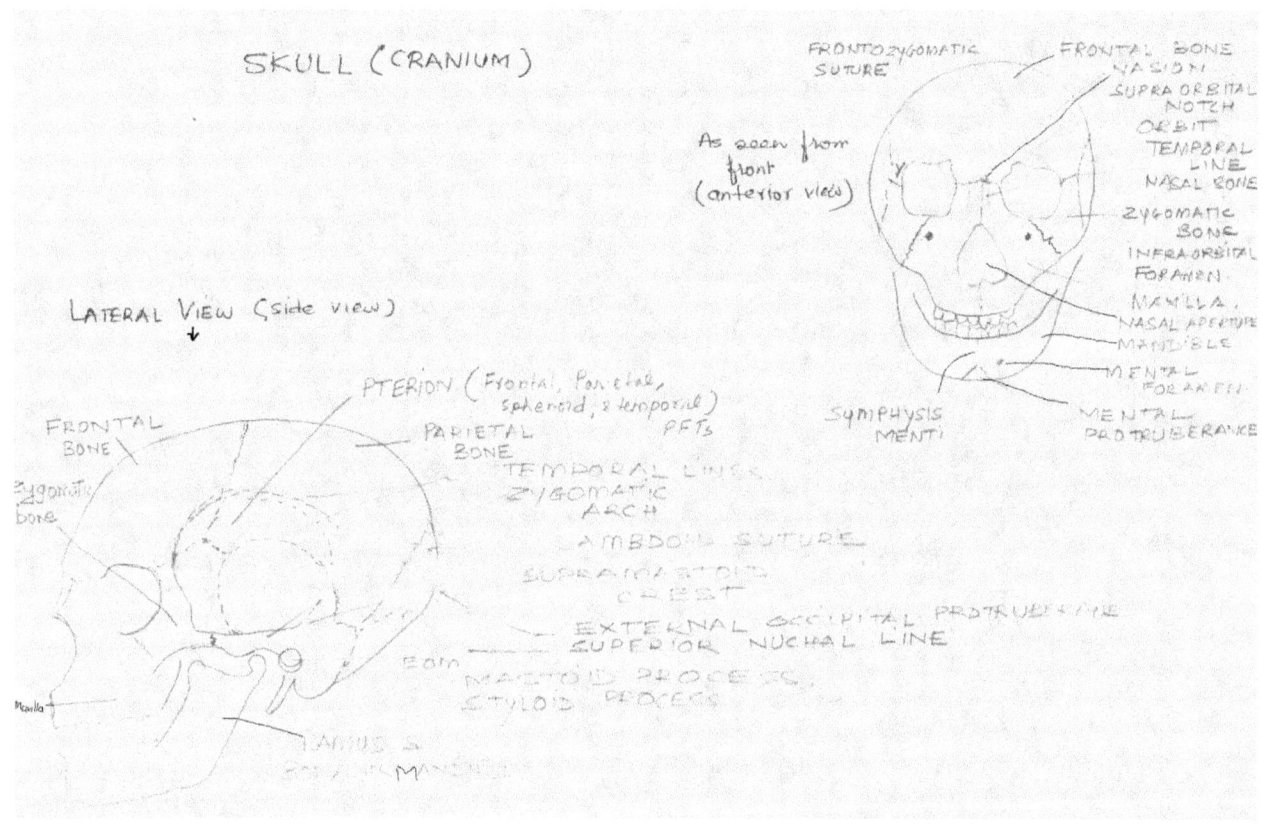

So, the first step is to see the skull. It is easy to identify frontal bone, parietal bone, temporal bone, occipital bone, orbit, and maxilla. locate nasal aperture in the frontal view. and pterion and zygomatic process in the lateral view of skull.

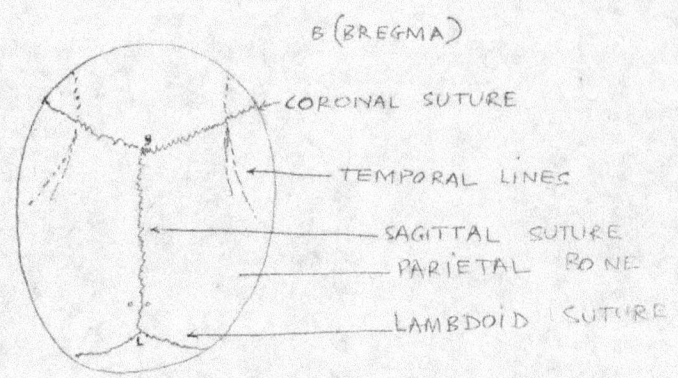

Skull As seen from above (Norma verticalis)

Coronal suture is placed between the frontal bone and the two parietal bones.

Sagittal suture is in the median plane between the two parietal bones.

Lambdoid suture lies posteriorly between the occipital and the two parietal bones.

Metopic suture is occasionally present (in about 3 to 8% individuals. It lies in the median plane & separates the two halves of the frontal bone.

VERTEX is the highest point on the sagittal suture.
BREGMA is the meeting point between the coronal & sagittal sutures.
Membranous gap in fetal skull called anterior fontanelle (closes at 1½ yrs of age)

Source: B.D. Chaurasia's Human Anatomy
Third Edition CBS Publishers, Delhi

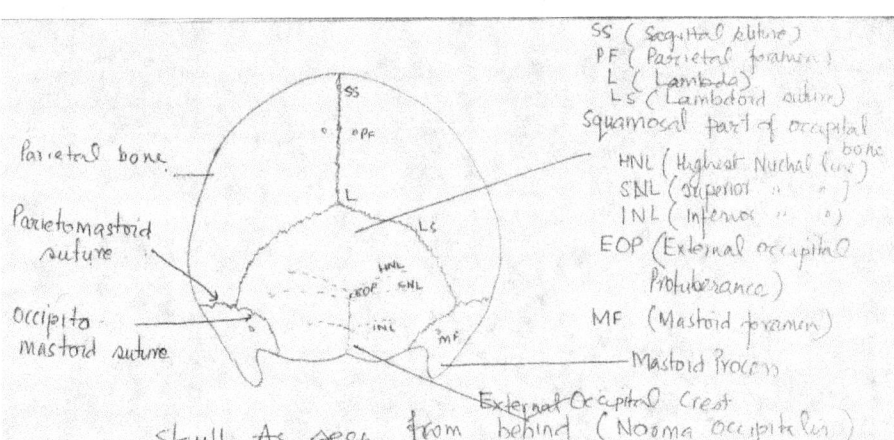

Skull as seen from behind (Norma Occipitalis)

SS (Sagittal suture)
PF (Parietal foramen)
L (Lambda)
LS (Lambdoid suture)
Squamosal part of occipital bone
HNL (Highest Nuchal line)
SNL (Superior " ")
INL (Inferior " ")
EOP (External Occipital Protuberance)
MF (Mastoid foramen)

Lambda is the meeting point between the sagittal and lambdoid suture. In the fetal skull this is the site of the posterior fontanelle which closes at 2 to 3 months of age.

The lambdoid suture lies between the occipital bone & the two parietal bones. Sutural bones are common along this suture.

The occipitomastoid suture lies between the occipital bone & the mastoid part of the temporal bone.

The parietomastoid suture lies between the parietal bone & the mastoid part of the temporal bone.

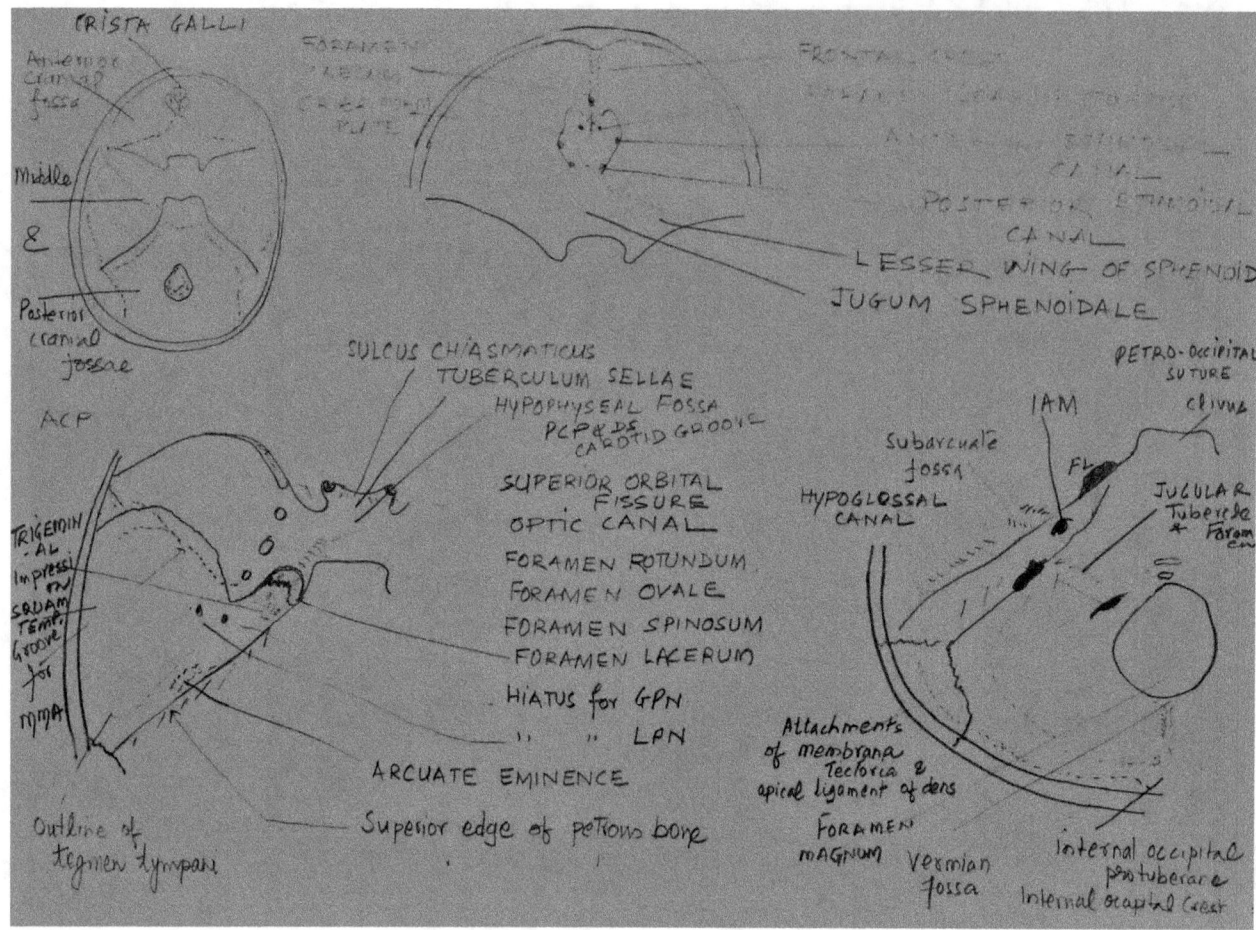

The first picture provides an idea about the three fossae of the inside of the cranium or skull. The anterior cranial fossa, middle cranial fossa and posterior cranial fossa. It is extremely important to know these three terms, as these three terms are frequently used by the experts in neuroanatomy and neurosurgery. This picture is a diagrammatic representation of the view of the skull base as seen from above after removing the skull cap. One should learn to draw this simple yet a very important diagram. Locate the greater wing of the sphenoid bone, anterior clinoid procees , petrous bone, posterior clinoid process and foramen magnum in this diagram. Rest of the three diagrams are are enlarged view of the base of the three intracranial fossae.

Just to make you aware about the inside of the cranium another simple diagram is drawn below . Identify and note the location of tent which divides inside the cranium into supratentorial and infratentorial compartments.

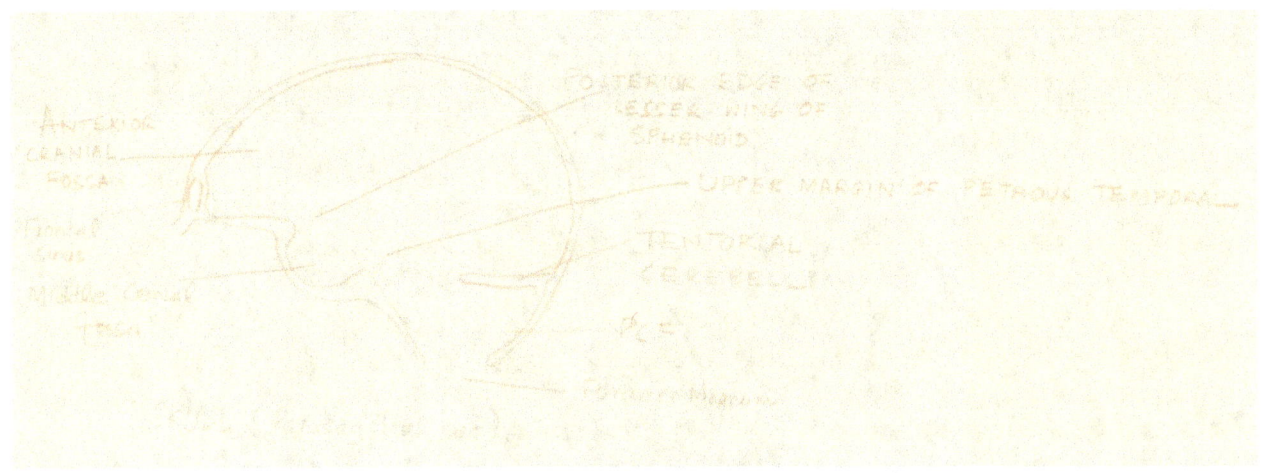

BRODMANN'S AREAS

As you know that almost all areas of the body are represented in the cerebral hemisphere which are known as Brodmann,s areas. These areas are given different numbers. Like Motor area, Sensory area, Speech area, visual area, hearing area.

Important functional areas of brain are :

Primary Motor area or Primary Motor Cortex or Motor Strip or Precentral Gyrus (area 4)

Primary Somatosensory cortex (areas 3,1,2 are situated in the post central gyrus, i.e. part of the Parietal lobe just posterior to the central sulcus)

Primary auditory area or Transverse gyrus of Heschl (areas 41 & 42)

Broca's Speech Area (area 44)is situated in the dominant inferior frontal gyrus which is usually left inferior frontal gyrus in right handed person.

Wernicke's area (Receptive speech area)

Frontal eye field (area 8)

Primary Visual Cortex (area 17)

Spinal cord is the caudal continuation of the medulla oblongata. When the distal part of brain stem is continued outside the foramen magnum it becomes the spinal cord. It is contained inside the vertebral canal formed inside the vertebral column. It is bounded anteriorly by the vertebral bodies and intervertebral discs and posteriorly by the lamina and spinous processes. The spinal nerves emerge from the intervertebral foramina.

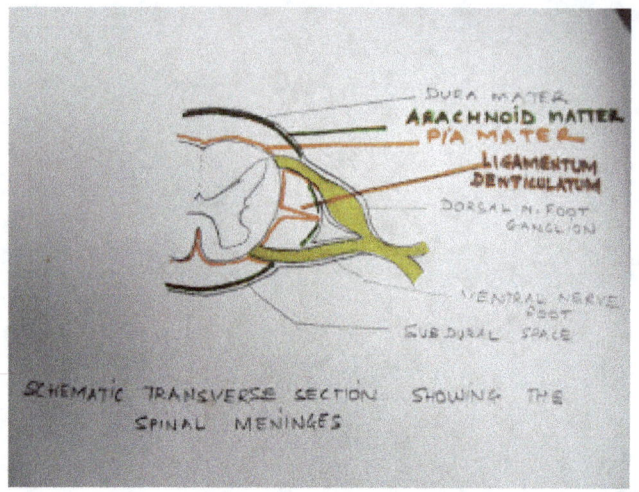

This is the schematic transverse section of the spinal cord. Spinal cord is also bounded by three meningeal layers as that of brain. Subarachnoid space contains CSF. Ligamentum denticulatum is the extension of the Piamater in spinal cord.

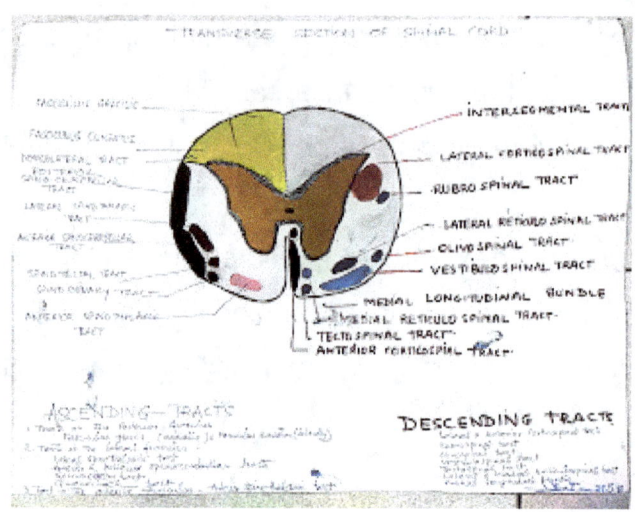

Role of Endoscopic Third Ventriculostomy (ETV) in treatment of Hydrocephalus

Now a days, the endoscopic treatment of hydrocephalus is an established technique of treating hydrocephalus. Previous works of Lespinase , Dandy , Mixter, Fay and Grant had contributed in the evolution of this concept.

Lespinasse in 1910 was the first one to perform endoscopic choroid plexus fulgration for treating hydrocephalus.

Dandy described the open technique for third ventriculostomy for treatment of hydrocephalus.

In 1923, Mixter first described percutaneous ventriculostomy, and Fay Grant published the visual record of endoscopic anatomy.

The aim of this surgery is to create a passage in the floor of the third ventricle and to allow the flow of CSF into the pre pontine cistern so that obstruction at the aqueduct can be avoided. The easiest example to explain is of obstructive hydrocephalus due to aqueductal stenosis. In this condition, patient presents with enlargement of the lateral ventricles and third ventricle. The obstruction at the aqueduct causes obstructive hydrocephalus and the cerebral sulci are effaced. So, an endoscope is introduced through the frontal horn of right lateral ventricle and advanced into the third ventricle through dilated Foramen of Monro. Floor of the third ventricle is visualized and an opening is made in the floor of the third ventricle allowing the CS flow to the pre-pontine cistern.

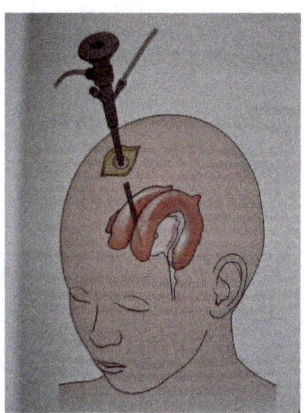

So, high success rate is seen in aqueductal stenosis and ventricular obstructions assosciated with tumors. Low success rate is expected in post tubercular hydrocephalus due to basal exudates at the basal cisterns and thickened third ventricular floor.

A variety of endoscopic equipments with some modification are available for neuroendoscopic procedures.

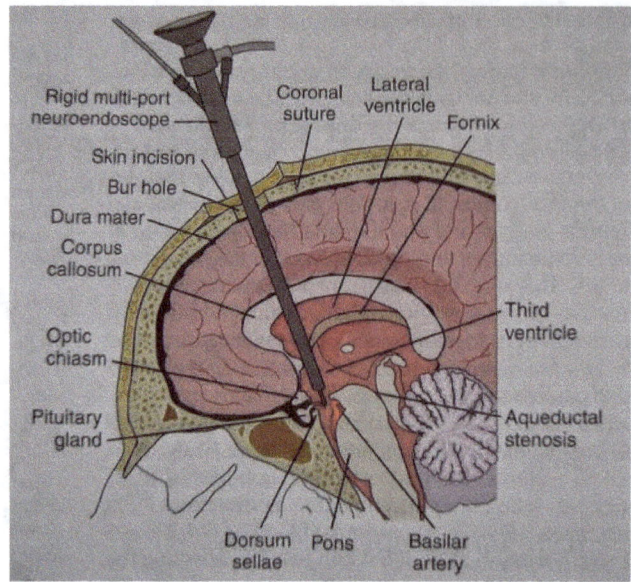

Endoscope is passed from right lateral ventricle to third ventricle through Foramen of Monro

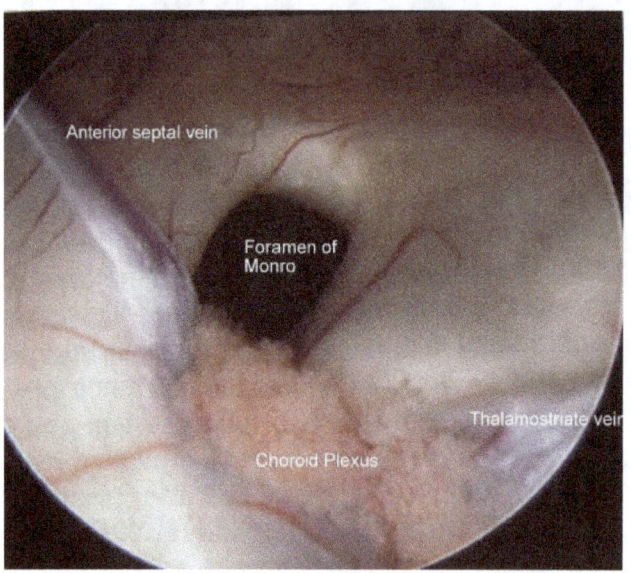

Intraoperative Endoscopic view of the structures at the Foramen of Monro

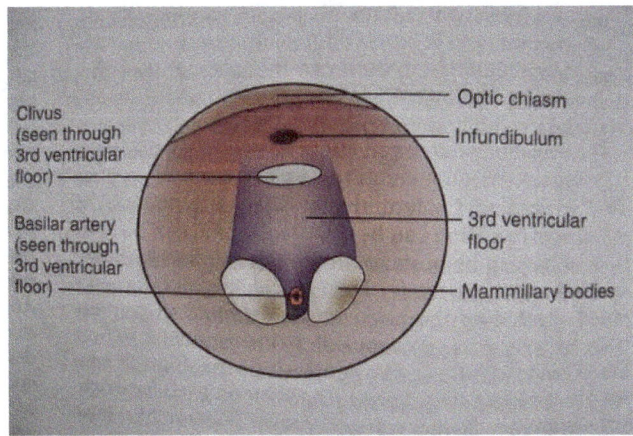

Diagrammatic depiction of the anatomical structures which are to be identified by the neurosurgeon

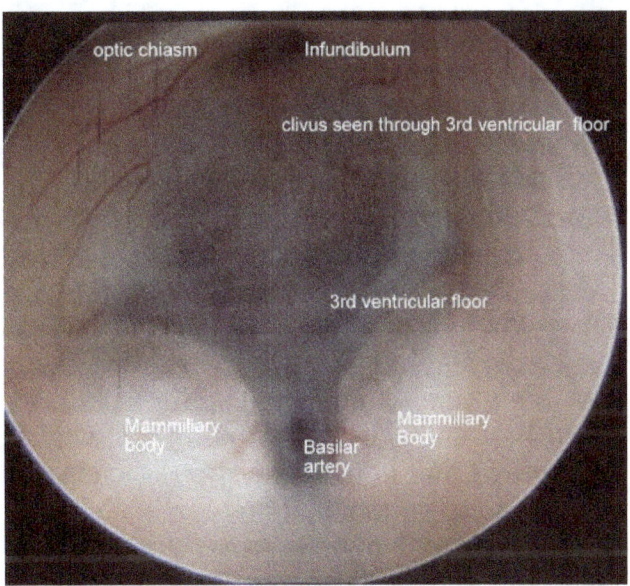

Intraoperative endoscopic view of the anatomical structures as seen at the floor of the third ventricle

Skull Base Neurosurgery in one page : Easy facts to develop insight

Every neurosurgical trainee should develop an insight about the nuances of skull base neurosurgery. If you are able to make a bur hole in skull, you have already taken first step in understanding and practicing skull base neurosurgery.

Aim of skull base neurosurgery is to reach deeper regions of the brain with minimal retraction of the brain tissue. Prolong retraction of brain parenchyma leads to edema, ischemia and brain damage and, in turn, increases post operative morbidity.

One should learn to draw the lateral view of skull depicting zygoma, pterion and orbit.

Fronto-temporal craniotomy or pterional craniotomy is very useful for approaching middle cranial fossa lesions. But this often requires prolong temporal lobe retraction, so adding orbito-zygomatic craniotomy makes the job easy. Therefore, little more work on skull base helps to reduce morbidity.

To understand the skull base surgery, one should know that cranial cavity can be divided into anterior, middle and posterior cranial fossa (learn to draw a line diagram showing ACF, MCF & PCF).

ACF floor can further be zoomed to see midline structures like crista galli, olfactory groove, planum sphenoidale and tuberculum sellae. Laterally roof of the orbit forms the floor of anterior cranial foosa (ACF). The anterior skull base tumors can be meningiomas (olfactory groove meningioma, planum sphenoidale meningioma or tuberculum sellae meningioma. For CSF rhinorrhea repair, excision & repair of intranasal encephalocele, exciosion of intracranial extension of ethenioneuroblastoma and excision of intracranial fungal granulomas extending into nasal cavity, and chordoma of the floor of the ACF, one should know bicoronal scalp inciosion, bifrontal craniotomy just above the orbit and anterior to the coronal suture, exteriorization of frontal air sinus, clipping and cutting of the superior sagittal sinus close to crista galli and opening the dura and retracting base of the frontal lobe backwards.

Mid sagittal image of the MRI is very easy to understand the relation of intracranial structures to the nasal cavity and how Trans nasal transphenoidal and transoral odondoidectomy is done. This image will also help you understand the supracerebellar infra tentorial approach for operating pineal tumor

.

Like usefulness of fronto temporal craniotomy for anteriorly placed lesions, midline sub occipital craniotomy is basic and of equal importance for operating lesions of midline posterior fossa structures. Scalp incision is made from external occipital protuberance to the C2 spinous process. Scalp is retracted and a bur hole is made in the occipital squama and the suboccipital craniectomy is done. Dura is opened in 'Y' shaped manner to avoid injury to the occipital sinus. Midline suoccipital craniectomy is done for operating Medulloblastoma, Cerebellar ependymoma, 4th ventricular tumor, posterior fossa decompression for Chiari malformation. If lesion is situated laterally like cerebellar astrocytoma the paramedian suboccipital craniectomy is done. far lateral, retromastoid cranectomy are done for other posterior fossa lesions.

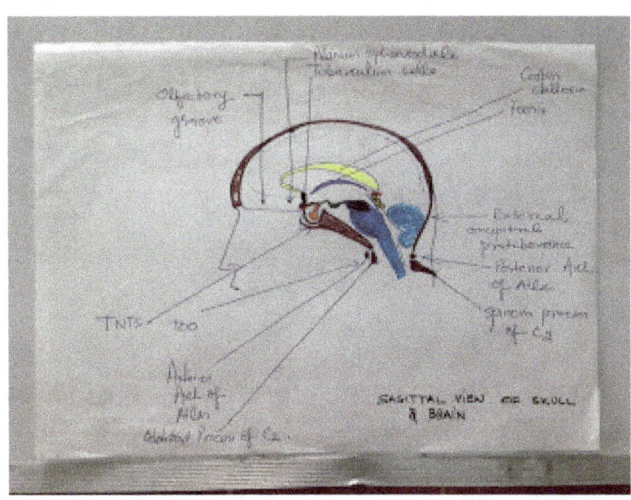

TNTS is abbreviation for for transnasal transsphenoidal surgery &
TOO stands for transoral surgery

In Fronto-temporal craniotomy, at the supraorbita ridge care should be taken to identify and preserve the supraorbital nerve and vessel passing through the supraorbital foramen or notch. These can be released with the aid of a chisel or drill. A bur hole is made at the McCarty keyhole. The sphenoid ridge is made as flat as possible down to the level of the meningo-orbital artery.

In orbital osteotomy , the peroorbita is separated from the roof of the orbit for a distance of 3 cm posteriorly from the supraorbital ridge, and it is also separated along the lateral wall of the orbit. A sagittal cut is made in the roof of the orbit from the cranial to the orbit side to a depth of at 3 cm posterior to the supraorbital ridge. A second cut is made above the zygomatic process of the frontal boneand extended posteriorly as deep as possible within the orbit. Third cut is a coronal cut made across the roof of the orbit to connect the previous cuts. In orbitozygomatic osteotomy, this coronal cut across the roof of the orbit extends laterally from the sagittal cut to the inferior orbital fissure. A third cut is made parallel to, but several millimeters above, the zygomaticomaxillary suture.

In Transbasal approach, after making the McCarty keyhole bilaterally, a bifrontal craniotomy is done as close to the floor of the frontal fossa as possible. The posterior wall of the frontal air sinus is removed and thereby cranializing the sinus.The medial floor of the frontal fossa, including the roof of the ethmoidal air cells, is removed . The lateral margins of the the bone removal are the medial walls of the orbit.
In Extended Transbasal approaches, a bone cut is made through the nasofrontal suture, sagittal cuts are made just medial to the supraorbital notch on each side. This allows en bloc removal of the central portion of the supraorbital bar.

Trans-sphenoidal approach is used for sellar lesions , especially pituitary adenoma, through nasal cavity.

In Anterolateral Extradural/ Intraduralapproach for cavernous sinus, after cranio-orbitozygomatic osteotomy, the optic canal is unroofed and its medial wall drilled. The superior orbital fissure should be u roofed and the anterior clinod process resected. The floor of the middle fossa between the SOF and the foramen rotundum is drilled and the foramen is enlarged. The middle meningeal artery is identified and followed to the foramen spinosum. It is coagulated and divided , thus allowing the dura to be elevated from the floor of the middle fossa. The dura is dissected in a lateral to medial fashion until the greater superficial petrosal nerve (GSPN) is encounterd.To avoid the risk of injury to the facial nerve, the GSPN is transected and the bone of the Glassock's triangle is drilled away, exposing the posterior loop of the ICA and freeing it from its bony canal to obtain proximal control. The dura is then ready for opening.

In Preauricular Subtemporal-Infratemporal approach, a temporal craniotomy is performed, temporal dura is stripped from the floor of the middle fossa and arcuate eminence is identified. This is the posterior extent of the dissection. The dural separation is then continued anteriorly to reach the foramen spinosum, where the MMA can be seen as it enters the cranial cavity. Zygomatic osteotomy is done. Anteriorly a V-shaped cut is made at the level of the frontozygomatic and zygomaticomaxillary suture. The posterior cut is made to include the condylar fossa. This cut is also V-shaped, with the apex of V just short of the foramen spinosum and the limbs spanning the anterior and posterior extent of the zygomatic root. V3 (mandibular) and V2 (maxillary) divisions of the fifth nerve then are exposed at the foramen ovale and rotundum, respectively. The GSPN may be cut close to the facial hiatus.

Transpetrosal approach include translabyrinthine and transcochlear approaches require division of the external ear canal and mastoidectomy.

Retrosigmoid craniotomy or craniectomy is used for surgery of cerebellopontine angle tumors. A retroauricular skin incision is made.

Midline or Paramedian suboccipital craniectomy is used for approaching posterior foassa lesion.

Extreme lateral approach is used for vertebral and vertebral- basilar junction aneurysm.

For approaching the posterior third ventricular lesions and Pineal tumors, supracerebellar infratentorial, occipital transtentrorial approach and interhemispheric approaches are useful.

Sources: Operative Neurosurgical anatomy by Damirez T. Fossett &Anthony J.Caputy (Thieme)

www.ingramcontent.com/pod-product-compliance
Lightning Source LLC
Chambersburg PA
CBHW082210220526

45470CB00010B/3110